When Girls Feel Fat

Helping Girls Through Adolescence

When Girls Feel Fat

Helping Girls Through Adolescence

Sandra Susan Friedman

FIREFLY BOOKS

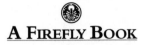

A FIREFLY BOOK

Published by Firefly Books Ltd. 2000

First Printing 2000

Cataloging-in-Publication Data
Friedman, Sandra Susan.
   When girls feel fat : helping girls through adolescence / Sandra Susan Friedman. - 2nd ed.
[   ] p. : cm.
Originally published: Toronto: HarperCollins, 1997.
Includes bibliographic references and index.

Summary : How to help adolescent girls with common problems of puberty, sexuality, body image, food and weight issues, and relationships.

ISBN 1-55209-517-7 (pbk.)

1. Child rearing. 2. Teenage girls. 3. Self-esteem in adolescence. 4. Body image in adolescence. I. Title.

305.23/ 55 -dc21   2000   CIP

Published in the United States in 2000 by
Firefly Books (U.S.) Inc.
P.O. Box 1338, Ellicott Station
Buffalo, New York, USA
14205

Design by Interrobang Graphic Design Inc.
Printed and bound in Canada by Friesens, Altona, Manitoba

Canadä

The Publisher acknowledges the financial support of the Government of Canada through the Book Publishing Industry Development Program for its publishing activities.

In loving memory of my parents,
Lottie and Louis Friedman

Contents

Acknowledgments

Many people helped make this book possible. I would like to thank Judy Chorney, Joyce Chorney, Susan Firus, Anne Stanley, Valerie Zwicher, Helga, Georgia, Lauriel, Megan and Madelaine, as well as all of the other mothers, fathers, mentors and girls who shared their experiences in groups, training workshops, counseling sessions, and in the course of friendship over the past years.

Thank you to my readers for their valuable insights and feedback. They include Carol Herbert, Margit McCorkle, Alisa Harrison, Louise Doyle, Carly McFetridge, Anne Carten, Ann Little, Daniel Schwartz, Patricia Schwartz, Lynn Sackville, Janice McDonough, Peter Hawes, Tom Barrett, Renalee Gore, Jonas Taub and Ruth Benedict.

I want to thank Dr. Lorna Medd for her continuous support of my work with girls and with eating disorder prevention; Marion Crook for her support as an author and a friend throughout the writing process; and Clea Sackville for giving me permission to include her personal experiences in this book. Booksellers Cathy Ellesmere and Nicki Breuer shared their expertise. Dan Liebman guided this book into production. My in-laws Dan and Margaret Fivehouse of Hawthorne, New Jersey, sent their love and encouragement.

Finally, I want to express my love and appreciation for my husband, friend and partner, Dan Fivehouse, for encouraging me to write this book, for the years he has spent as my sounding board, and for his superb job of editing not only this manuscript but also everything else that I write.

Introduction

One recent evening, I attended a pot luck dinner for mothers and daughters hosted by a friend and her twelve-year-old daughter. As we worked our way through each other's culinary contributions, we talked about ourselves and our concerns.

We shared our personal experiences as the evening progressed, as women and girls often tend to do. We ate good food and laughed a lot, and learned things about each other that we really didn't know before. The girls were eager to contribute to the discussion, to share their opinions and have their voices heard.

While there were variety and diversity in our experiences, there was also a common thread. Regardless of our different ages and interests, we all had times when we *felt fat*. Whenever we were unable to express our feelings directly or talk about the things that were really important to us, we turned them against ourselves and encoded them in a *language of fat*. We felt fat when we were angry, fat when we were lonely, and we felt fat when we had no other way of expressing our feelings and concerns.

The mothers talked mostly about the changes that their daughters were going through during puberty. They expressed their hopes and fears for them during adolescence and as they entered the adult world. They were worried about their daughters' safety. They worried that their daughters would begin to tune them out and that their relationships with them would become strained. They worried that their daughters would lose their sense of themselves and begin to be overly concerned with how they looked and with pleasing other people. They worried about eating disorders, which are rampant, as well as the other health and social risks that girls face. Most of all, they worried that despite their best intentions, they would end up doing something wrong. They bombarded me with questions about the work I was doing, and asked me for strategies to keep their lines of communication open.

This book is about the lives and experiences of girls and women. It's about what happens to us when we go through puberty and begin to worry about our weight and to lose connection with ourselves. Examining how girls begin worrying about their weight provides a key to opening discussion about what happens to girls in the process of growing up female in a male world. This book looks at girls' development and at the risks they face as they grow up. It provides us with skills to communicate better with girls and to decode the messages that lie underneath the times when girls feel fat. In helping girls delve beneath the surface and in learning more about their world, we sometimes stir up old feelings in ourselves and bring up issues of our own. And because we as women bring our personal selves into whatever we do, this book is not just about girls. It is also about us.

When Girls Feel Fat is primarily addressed to mothers and other female mentors who work with and care about girls. It is written from a woman's perspective and is about our issues and our lives. I have written this book from a female perspective because that is what I know. I realize this is somewhat unfair to fathers because parenting should be a partnered exercise, as more men are coming to accept.

It is my hope that fathers and other male mentors will also read this book. Men influence girls' development through the ways they act toward girls, in their attitudes concerning adult women, in their feelings about fathering, in their experiences with their own parents, and in the kinds of male/female relationships they maintain in the world. Fathers play a significant role in determining how girls feel about themselves and their abilities, and in the kinds of relationships that girls will ultimately have with other men.

As a father or male mentor, learning what it is like to be female will enhance your relationships with your wife and daughters and with other women and girls. You might find that you can relate to some of the experiences in the book and can apply the information to yourself. Where your experience differs because of your gender, looking at what it was like to grow up male might help you learn about yourself and provide you with insights into your behavior and your attitudes.

How This Book Came About

This book is the culmination of my thirty years of working with girls and women that began when I was an elementary school teacher who had an uneasy relationship with food and weight. I taught my way up into high school before I left teaching in 1976. Later, as an MA student in psychology, I was able to explore the issues that I had been deflecting onto my body, and I learned skills for dealing with concerns about my weight. In 1980, I went into private practice as a therapist and also worked in partnership with Doris Maranda to develop and facilitate groups for women.

Over time, we progressed from being "fat therapists" into "eating disorder specialists" as the numbers of young women with anorexia and bulimia began to grow. While our clients and group participants kept changing, the dynamics and concerns remained the same. Underneath the bingeing and purging and dieting and fasting are the stories of women's everyday lives. Feeling fat has little to do with body size. It is an encoded way of talking about what it is like to be a woman in a world that is defined by and for men.

In the 1990s, my professional life came full circle. Shifting the focus of my work to prevention, I was given an opportunity to develop an eating disorder prevention program for girls. I knew that worrying about weight is a universal part of growing up female. I decided that if we were going to keep this preoccupation from developing into eating disorders, we had to address the issue just at the point when young girls began to feel fat.

My program *Just for Girls* is an open discussion group that looks at what happens to girls as they reach puberty in a society that encourages them to define themselves by the numbers on the scale. The program teaches girls to recognize *when* they feel fat (and ugly and stupid) and encourages them to tell the stories that are encoded underneath. The group facilitators validate the girls' experiences and provide them with a context for why they felt the way they did. *Just for Girls* soon became a prototype for programs that deal with girls. I began to get phone calls from mothers who wanted something more specific and comprehensive for their own use. Like the mothers at my friends' dinner, they wanted skills they could learn and strategies they could try with their own girls at home.

I have talked to many mothers in the course of writing this book. I've drawn stories from my private practice and from women that I know. I've worked with girls in groups and interacted with them in their classrooms. Throughout this book you will hear about their experiences. Most of the voices are individual people. Some are composites that were put together to illustrate how many women and girls feel. While I have changed their names to respect their privacy, the honesty and integrity of their feelings remain.

How to Use This Book

Think of *When Girls Feel Fat* as a kind of partnership. I provide you with stories and information, skills to use and suggestions to try – which I hope will be helpful. You bring your own life experiences and your relationships with girls. No matter how much information I give you, you are the best authority on your daughter and on the other girls in your life. You don't have to become perfect or make major changes in your life to benefit from this book. You just have to be open and willing to try different things.

When Girls Feel Fat is made up of four sections. "Setting the Stage" provides the framework for the book. It introduces you to the subject of gender and describes female development through early adolescence. It looks at why girls lose their sense of self as they grow up and learn to encode their experiences in a language of fat. You might be tempted to skip this section and go straight to the "how to" section of the book. If you do so, please come back and read it at another time. You will find that you learn a lot about yourself.

"Building Our Skills" explains how girls can become preoccupied with food and weight and can develop an eating disorder if we do not intervene. It looks at the true feelings of girls who feel fat, and at the *grungies* – a term coined to describe the negative things we tell ourselves. This section provides you with the skills to help girls decode their grungies so that they don't get so caught up in the language of fat. You will see how you as a mother, father, or other mentor can maintain your ties with girls through adolescence. It helps you become aware of your own emotional baggage that sometimes gets in the way. The chapter on communication teaches you new skills and/or enhances those that you already have.

"Putting Our Skills to Work" takes you more intimately into the world of girls. It gives you background information on their concerns and encourages you to practice your new skills. The "Time Out" in each chapter is designed to teach you more about yourself, while "Time with Each Other" suggests exercises that you and the girls in your life can try together. Finally, "Resources" lists books and videos if you want to know more about a certain topic and programs that might interest you.

As you read this book, I hope you find parts where you agree with me and relate to what I've written. Some of this information may be new to you or you may wonder where I am coming from. You may find that in some areas your experience and knowledge are greater than mine or find that you disagree with my point of view. That is all right. You are the best judge of what is valuable to you. Use the parts you agree with or think will be helpful. Leave out the ones that make you uncomfortable and just go on from there. The strategies and suggestions in this book are just that: suggestions. Not all of them will be of use to every reader. Pick and choose the ones that you relate to best and adapt them to your own style. If something doesn't work the first time, repeat it again or try a different approach. Remember that there is no perfect way of being a mother or mentor, and that there is no right or wrong way to do this work.

I hope you enjoy this book and that while you are reading it, you will find parts that make you laugh. I hope you and your special girl will grow together and that you will open up new doors. Most of all, I hope you have fun and learn to trust yourself.

SETTING THE STAGE

■

Entering the World of Girls

1

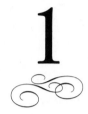

Gender

The Telephone Story

When I first met my husband, we lived in different neighborhoods. We spent a lot of time talking on the telephone, as part of the process of getting to know one another. Dan would call me every evening and ask me about my day. I would obligingly provide him with a blow-by-blow account that included not only a description of what I did, but also a detailed account of just about every human interaction that I had. Inevitably there would come a point in the conversation where I would feel myself becoming anxious because of silence at the other end of the line.

"Are you listening?" I would ask the silent receiver in my hand.

"Yes, yes, go on," he would say. And so I would continue until once again I would be stopped by his seeming lack of response.

"Are you still listening?" I would ask again.

"Yes, yes, go on," he would reply.

At some point in the conversation I would begin to hesitate in what I was saying because I began to feel what I perceived was distance between us. It seemed that no matter how much we wanted to communicate with each other, we would get caught up in a dynamic that left us both frustrated. Years later, when I began to study female development, the pieces finally fell into place and I learned how these communication differences come about.

Women talk to make each other feel part of one another's lives. We share the details, we make noises to provide empathy and support – to let the other person know how we feel. When we speak to each other, we know that the other person is alive and interacting with us. We emphasize the process of communication more than the goal.

Men grow up with a different perception of the world. They wait to hear the whole story to the end so that they can unravel the problem and tell you what to do to solve it.[1] When I look back now, I realize that the longer I took in getting to what Dan felt was the point of the conversation, the harder it was for him to figure out what response was necessary from him. The more intently he listened so as not to miss the crucial facts, the more silent he became.

What he did not seem to understand was that I didn't require any particular solution; all that I required was an interactive response – *any* response. In turn, I was put off by his thoughtful silence. I felt all the more anxious and frustrated. While he felt he was being a considerate listener, I did not get the feedback that I needed in order to feel heard. We eventually learned that we were dealing with two very different and gender-oriented styles of communication.

A Tale of Two Cultures

I have chosen to begin this book by telling this story because it opens the door to understanding how men and women make up two separate cultures – with quite different languages and different ways of interpreting and responding to the world. We need to understand these cultural differences in order for us to address what happens to girls as they grow up, and why so many girls inevitably feel fat.

From the moment we are born we begin the process of learning how to fit ourselves into our society. We need to know what is expected of us in order for us to get along with others and to be part of a community. We need to know about the attitudes and values that are part of our particular culture, and about the kinds of behaviors that are acceptable, as well as those that are not. We learn these things through the process of socialization, which teaches us how to become social beings.

The factor of gender – whether we are female or male – plays a major part in shaping our lives. Gender socialization teaches us how to act and behave separately as women or as men, and defines the different roles that we are then expected or required to play. It determines what we are named, how we are treated, what clothes we wear, what toys we are given and what games we play. As we mature, gender socialization influences the kinds of job choices we have and the amount of money that we get paid for our work.

Gender socialization begins at birth and continues throughout our lives. As soon as a pregnancy is confirmed, future parents begin to fantasize about their baby. Their dreams are influenced by their own experiences, by their particular culture and by the society in which we all live. For many expectant fathers, a son will be someone to do things with. For mothers, a daughter will be someone to be close to. Few parents will envision a daughter who will quarterback the Pittsburgh Steelers, or a son who will excel as a daycare worker in an inner city school.

Right from the beginning girls and boys tend to march to different drummers. In the hospital nursery their parents tend to "see" girls as smaller, finer-featured, softer and less alert than their brothers, who are "seen" as being hardier and stronger.[2] Once at home, girls will be treated differently than boys.[3] Many mothers tend to touch their infant sons more often and provide them with more active stimulation, especially when they cry. When girls cry, the response is different. Girls are cuddled and soothed and calmed down.[4]

As babies grow up, their parents have different expectations of them and provide them with different kinds of learning situations that will teach them gender-appropriate behavior and help them realize gender-specific goals. It is common for parents to be more strict and demanding with their sons than they are with their daughters. They expect their sons to achieve more in the world, and they encourage and reward them for being independent, competitive and responsible. They also give them more freedom to explore. Boys are given toys such as trucks, building blocks, tools and sports equipment, which are meant to encourage inventiveness, exploration and manipulation. As they grow up, many of their activities are action-oriented. They are taught to do and make things, and figure things out for themselves.[5]

Girls are expected to remain physically and emotionally close to their parents. They are praised for being nurturing, understanding, compliant, cooperative and – most especially – pretty. Girls are given dolls, cradles, strollers, kitchens and stuffed animals, which teach them to nurture and take care of others. Drawing, painting and sewing encourage a more passive creativity than the kind offered to boys. Girls are watched over and protected and are more restricted in their activities. When they have a problem, their mothers often tend to solve it for them instead of encouraging them to figure it out on their own. Though they don't intend to do so, mothers often end up instilling a sense of learned helplessness in girls.[6]

When children enter the school system, the gender socialization begun by their parents is institutionalized, a process that I will return to later in this book. Factors such as race, ethnicity and socioeconomic class also reinforce differing standards of behavior and expectations for girls and boys (and, later on, for women and men). Relatives, friends, child care workers, employers, religious institutions and the media also exert their various powerful influences.

Trying to Narrow the Gender Gap

Some people think that we can narrow the gender gap and ameliorate the effects of gender socialization if we teach girls competitive sports, give them trucks to play with, and take guns away from boys and encourage them to play with dolls. It doesn't happen quite that way, however.

Nick and Lynn have tried to soften the extremes of gender socialization by raising their daughter, Clea, in an environment that is as diverse and gender-neutral as possible. They both parent, they both cook and they both work as professionals outside the home. The family rarely watches television and when they do it's usually public broadcasting or rental videos. Clea has been given a whole range of toys and activities to experience. By the time she was five, she was quite proficient on the family computer.

Thus when Clea showed me her Christmas wish list that year, I was taken aback. She asked for a Mary Poppins Barbie, a full-size Barbie, a Barbie house, an Ariel Barbie, a bubbling Barbie, a Kitty Surprise, a Bunny Surprise, a real cat, a Liddle Kiddie, a Kelly doll with stroller, a Chickie surprise, a wine glass horse, a little pet shop, a bus for Kelly, a Cinderella coach and a remote control car.

"She also plays with trucks," said Lynn, "but when she does, the big truck is the daddy truck, the next size is the mommy truck, and the little ones are baby trucks!"

Little girls will always find something to relate to. Little boys will inevitably make a fist, extend their index fingers and say "bang, bang." Trying to make girls and boys the same does not begin to address the fundamental differences in the ways in which they experience and respond to the world.

UNDERSTANDING GENDER DIFFERENCES

There was a time when society thought that all human beings developed in much the same way. The results of medical research performed on men were routinely applied to women because it was thought that aside from their sex organs, their bodies were the same. Just about every course in Psych 101 or Human Development emphasized the psychoanalytic theory of Sigmund Freud and the psychosocial theory of Erik Erikson – both of whom positioned men as the norm. When certain medical treatments didn't work, and when most girls and women came out second best on the developmental scales, we never questioned that something was wrong with our dependence upon these theories, but took it for granted that something was wrong with us as women. For many years, we accepted the myth that we were inferior and limited our expectations of ourselves. When we tried to be equal to men, we worked hard to make ourselves the same as them.

In the past twenty years, we have begun to gather evidence that shows that while men and women are similar in many ways, we are not the same. Studies show that in addition to differences in socialization, there are profound gender differences in biology and psychology. We have begun to recognize that even when women and men as individuals do the exact same things, we will most likely experience and describe them differently.

Despite the ongoing debate over whether gender differences are biological, psychological or learned through experience, few people will disagree that these differences do exist. Yet not every man or every woman falls neatly into every single gender category. As you continue reading, you might say to yourself, "Wait a minute, I know men who are nurturing and women who are very competitive. My daughter fights with her friends, but my son gets along fine with his. I know girls who do fabulously well in math and boys who are terrible at science. What about them? They don't fit into the picture that you are describing." It is important to remember that in writing in generalities I am not writing about single individuals, but about statistically significant groups of men and groups of women who have certain things in common and exhibit certain differences as a class.

Height is a good example of how such generalities work. If we look at a large number of people, we find that on the whole the men are taller than the women – even though some women would be taller than some men. We, as individuals, are all different. But we share groups of characteristics that are common to our sex.

Understanding gender differences gives us a better appreciation of our own uniqueness and a context for our behavior. It helps us avoid the misunderstandings that occur when society makes the assumption that men and women see the world through the same eyes and decides that those who do not share the dominant point of view are inferior or wrong.

Studies that look at differences in hormonal makeup and in brain structure (which address how we acquire our identities) and studies that teach us about gender socialization all contribute to a composite of male or female characteristics that describes the opposite ends of a continuum of human behavior. A continuum is a path that describes how things progress. This continuum describes all the possible combinations of male/female characteristics. It lets us understand how it is that there are things that we label as "male" that apply to women and things that we label as "female" that apply to men.

This continuum is also influenced by environment, culture, early childhood experiences, our position in our families and the numbers of brothers and sisters that we have. We need to have a context for the values that we assign to the skills, traits and behaviors associated with being male or female. And we need to know how these differences influence the course of our lives.

Biology: It's How We're Made

When the sperm fertilizes the ovum at conception, the child-to-be inherits twenty-three pairs of chromosomes. Each pair has one chromosome from the mother and one from the father. These chromosomes carry the genetic blueprint for reproducing a human being. They also carry specific traits from the parents' ancestors that may be passed on to the child. The twenty-third set of chromosomes (sex chromosomes) determines whether the child-to-be will be a girl or a boy. The mother contributes one X-shaped chromosome. The father donates either an X or a Y. If an X-bearing sperm fertilizes the ovum at conception, the XX combination will produce a female fetus. If a Y-bearing sperm gets there first, the XY combination will produce a fetus that contains the programming to become male.

According to Anne Moir and David Jessel, authors of *Brain Sex: The Real Difference between Men and Women*,[7] for the first few weeks after conception every fetus is female. At about six weeks of gestation, a fetus that is genetically male (XY) develops special cells that produce the male hormones or androgens, the main one being testosterone. These hormones stimulate the development of male genitalia. They also change the basic pattern and structure of the brain. Boys receive several massive doses of male hormones – first at six weeks of conception when their brains are beginning to take shape, and then again in puberty to kick-start their sexuality. The greater the concentration of male hormone the fetus is exposed to, the closer the adult male will be to the male end of the continuum of human behavior. The lesser amount of male hormone, the more his behavior will tend to the female end of the continuum.

The same process holds true for girls. In the fetus that begins genetically XX, the reproductive organs continue to develop along female lines. Tiny amounts of testosterone in the ovaries influence the developing brain and are a necessary part of its development. If the fetus inadvertently receives a large dose of testosterone at a certain point in its development in the womb, the brain structure will be altered, and the way the girl perceives and interacts with the world will be more masculine.

According to psychologist Dr. June Reinisch, director of the Kinsey Institute in Ohio, we are all "flavored by our prenatal chemical development. The amount of male hormone we receive and when we receive it contributes to a continuum of behaviors that include aggressively competitive athletic girls, and boys who are preoccupied with clothes and dolls. It determines which girls are better than others in math, and which boys are less aggressive and more cooperative in nature than other boys."[8]

Moir and Jessel believe that it is differences in brain structure that contribute to the differences in perceptions, priorities and behaviors in the sexes. Male brains are more specialized than female ones. The left side is almost exclusively set aside for the control of verbal abilities including speaking, writing, reading and language. The right side controls visual abilities including spatial relations and abstract thought.

The female brain is different. It is more diffuse. The functional division between the left and right sides of the brain is less clearly defined. Both sides are used in verbal activities and both sides are used in visual activities.[9] (A cautionary note: most of the popular books written about the "left brain/right brain" concept reference the male brain only!)

Many of the differences between girls and boys begin in utero and are evident shortly after birth. There is a tendency for girls to be more interested in people, and boys to be more interested in things. For example, studies of babies who are two to four days old show that girls spend almost twice as long maintaining eye contact with adults. They are more tuned in to facial expressions and emotional nuances and will lose interest once the connection is broken. At four months, most girls can distinguish between photographs of people they know and those of strangers. The female brain responds more intensely to emotion. Feelings, especially sadness, activate neurons in an area eight times larger in the female brain than in the male. Even before they can understand language, girls seem to be better at identifying the emotional content of speech.[10] Girls are more sensitive to touch and more sensitive to their environment than boys. They react more readily to loud noises and to cold and dampness.

For boys, the interpersonal connection is less important than the activity. Boy babies will continue to jabber away at toys and objects in their cribs long after the adult has ended the contact. Boys are more active and wakeful than girls. They are more sensitive to bright light and focus more on depth perception and perspective than on the wider picture.[11]

What makes girls and boys better at different things seems to be the degree to which a particular area of the brain is specifically devoted to a particular activity – whether it is focused or diffuse. Girls learn to speak earlier because they have more efficient brain organization for speech. Their skill at verbal memory helps them master grammar and the intricacies of language. Boys outnumber girls four to one in classes for remedial reading, stuttering and speech defects.

Boys have better hand/eye coordination. They are more able to manipulate objects in space. Later on, they are better at interpreting maps, solving mazes, and doing the kinds of mathematics that involve abstract concepts of space, relationships and theory.[12]

It is important to remember that neither brain structure is "superior" to the other. Nor are girls and boys restricted in what they can do because of the structure of their brains. However, because parts of the male brain grow at times and rates different from the corresponding parts of the female brain, girls and boys may not develop the same skills at the same time in their development.[13] As well, the ways in which they learn these skills and perform these tasks are different.

Psychology: *It's All How You Feel*

In the past twenty years, research in female development has shown us that there are profound differences between boys and girls in the ways that their identities are formed and in how their sense of self is developed. Male development is based on an assumption that in order to grow up you have to separate from your parents and learn to do things on your own.[14] You have to become an individual, stand on your own two feet and be your own man.

The psychological theories that describe boys and men tend to see their development as taking place in progressive or hierarchical stages. Once you complete one stage, you rise to the next one. Each stage reinforces the qualities and abilities that you mastered before and teaches you new ones that are considered to be increasingly more appropriate and mature. In Erikson's psychosocial theory, for example, if you have difficulty learning trust you'll have a harder time with autonomy, which comes next.[15]

Because society encourages boys to separate from their mothers at a very early age, and because relatively few fathers are involved in the immediate care of their children, most boys grow up having no one with whom to develop lasting emotional connections. Boys develop a sense of "self-in-separation,"[16] which is based on accomplishment – on how well they perform out in the world. Intimacy, and the ability to form relationships, does not enter into the male developmental scheme until boys reach adolescence. Thus, for many boys, it tends to be intertwined with (and sometimes inseparable from) sexuality.

Girls develop differently, according to Janet L. Surrey and her colleagues at the Wellesley College Center for Research on Women. Female development is based upon the increasing ability to build and enlarge mutually enhancing relationships.[17] Girls develop their identity or sense of self in the context of their relationships. This is where they learn to recognize their connection to and separateness from the other.[18]

From birth, the emphasis is on the dynamic relationship between mother and child that continues and becomes more complex as girls grow up. Instead of a "self-in-separation," girls develop a "self-in-relation."[19] This evolves through a process that begins in infancy with the interaction between mother and daughter. The relationship deepens as girls develop an ability to experience emotion and a growing capacity for empathy with others. It then moves on into a conscious adult response which involves an awareness of the mechanics of a relational process that empowers both people.[20]

Because relationship and identity are intertwined, girls grow up to be interdependent. They learn to evaluate situations not only in terms of their individual responses, but also within the context of whatever others may be involved.[21] They are not only concerned with their own individual well-being but also with the well-being of those systems in which they participate.

Language: It's What You Say as Well as How You Say It

As babies grow into toddlers and begin to talk, they learn about male and female social roles through the different ways in which language is used and through other rituals that make up communication. Language is a major part of culture and is an important way of passing along and reinforcing our traditions, principles and beliefs. Language socialization occurs in two ways. When children interact with adults, they learn that women speak differently to women and girls than they do to men and boys. They also talk about different things. The same holds true for men.[22] When children play with other children of the same sex, they learn to use the respective language and reinforce the speaking rituals common to their gender.[23]

Language operates in a dynamic fashion for boys. Male language is logical and is based on reason. It serves as a way for them to exert power over others and/or to keep people from pushing them around. It is a very effective tool in winning arguments and for challenging and/or deflecting other people. It establishes the boy in a secure hierarchical niche by keeping other people a safe distance away.[24]

Language has an entirely different structure and function for girls. They use language and the process of talking as a means to draw people closer to them and to establish connections between them. Sounds, gestures and body language are used to deepen intimacy and to show rapport and understanding. Sharing is a way of holding relationships together, of involving the other person in their life.[25]

Girls also use language to create and maintain equality between each other. Adult women use the same rituals, even if they are not equal in status. "Trouble talk"[26] is a way of ensuring that one person will not have more power than the other. It works like this: if I tell you that I have a problem and you tell me what to do, then you're up (and have the power) and I'm down. This is primarily how boys interact with one another. But if I have a problem and you say "Oh yeah, I know what you mean. The same thing happened to me" and then you share a similar situation of your own, we're still equal – even if you give me advice. In later chapters, we'll look at how to integrate trouble talk into our relationships with girls.

Play: Learning to Be in the World

Once children reach the age of two or three they begin to play mostly with other children of the same sex. When boys play with each other their activities tend to be centered around doing physical things. Regardless of whether they play or watch, team sports teach them about competition, about the importance of rules, about winning and losing, about being the best – being on top. Not everybody is equal in the games that boys play. There are boys at the top and boys at the bottom – the hot stars and the average joes. The hot stars at the top are usually good or exceptional athletes. They give orders and push the average joes around.[27]

Boys continually measure themselves against each other in order to figure out where they stand in relation to one another. Because boys consider it important to be respected for their abilities, having someone tell them what to do implies that they do not measure up to the task. They interpret this as a loss of status and a lack of confidence in them.

When girls play, their games are based on communication and connection and on taking turns. Girls play in small groups that concentrate on the interactions between them. In games such as skipping and hopscotch, the competition between girls is indirect. The emphasis is not on being the best but rather on being included, something that is really important to girls.[28]

When girls are about eight or nine, they begin to learn that friends not only play together but they also help one another. They learn that friendships have a certain give-and-take. Around puberty, their friendships become more mutual. Girls begin to participate in ongoing, committed relationships that demand more of them than just doing things for each other. They are possessive of each other – because it takes a long time to make a close friend, and it's painful when she wants to make other friends, too. In order to feel secure, girls need to know how vulnerable they can be with one another – how much of themselves they can reveal. They continually check each other out to see how close and how distant they are from the other person. Underlying their interactions are the questions: "Do you love me?" and "What do I need to do to maintain the connection with you?"[29]

Conflict: I Want It, You Have It

Psychologist Amy Sheldon studied preschool boys and girls in the University of Minnesota Child Care Center. She found that conflict had different meanings for boys and girls. Conflict was a natural part of the way that boys played.[30] They tended to argue more than girls over objects. They fought with one another and tended to pursue their own goals. They were more physical with each other and tried to get their own way by dominating one another. When Tony and Nick both wanted the toy telephone, Nick resolved the conflict by taking the telephone by force.

Sheldon found that sometimes boys would fight as a way of entering into play. Just at the point where you want to break them up, suddenly they're best friends. As boys get older, conflict becomes a major part of their games – especially in team sports. Boys learn to bond with each other in an "us-against-them" scenario. Nowhere is this better seen than in professional team sports when someone scores a goal. But as the composition of the team changes, so do the loyalties.[31]

Girls' conflicts tend not to last as long as boys'. Girls tend to balance their own interests with those of the other girls. Rather than confront one another directly, girls will find subtle ways of showing disapproval. They will stop playing with each other or change the game rather than fight.[32] When girls can't resolve the situation through negotiation, threatening to exclude the other person ("You can't come to my birthday party") is much more effective than physical force. As girls get older they continue to handle conflict in a way that preserves the connection between them. Their games generally don't have as many rules. If someone is going to be left out or hurt, or if there are other mitigating circumstances, girls will break the rules or change them to accommodate the situation. As the chapter on friends will show, however, there is a dark side to girls' friendships. When girls do break the connection between them, it is usually through exclusion and through verbal rather than physical aggression.

Putting It into Practice

These pictures that I have painted for you are composites of male and female cultures. You may relate to only some of the parts yourself. You may see people that you know in others. No matter where we fit on the continuum of human behavior, we are influenced by our particular gender culture. It gives us a unique perspective on our world. It plays a major role in how we learn, in the stories we tell (and in the ways in which we tell them), in what we think is important and in how we get things done.

Just as men learn to do things on their own as independent entities, we women grow ever more interdependent. Just ask yourself, how many girls does it take to go to the bathroom? Two, since we usually travel in pairs. What do women talk about? Mostly relationships. Every time I pass two women on the street or sit next to women in a restaurant, I catch fragments of conversation that include, "And he said/she said …" How many women does it take to solve a problem? Two or three depending on the size of the problem. We solve problems and make decisions by talking things through, and the size of the problem determines how many friends we phone. Sharing reassures us that we are not alone in what we feel and that we have a right to feel what we are feeling. It allows us to ask for and receive feedback and to experiment with different solutions. When women address problem solving, we first go through a process of establishing all conceivable alternatives before we make up our minds.

The way we speak to one another and what we say ensures that we remain equal and are thus able to balance the intimacy or connection between us. We engage with one another on many levels. We provide each other continuously with clues as to how we feel through our body language, and through the empathic sounds we make. We make ritual noises and say things such as "ahah," "hmm," and "I know how you feel. That must be terrible!" We nod our heads and lean in toward one another. We interrupt each other to make sure we understand the details, to interject our own point of view, to share our experiences and to validate those of the other person.

When people withdraw from us, or don't respond, or when only one of us gets to speak, the rhythm of communication is interrupted and the connection between us is broken. We feel anxious when that happens. Sometimes we blame the other person. Often we deal with our anxiety by blaming ourselves or by trying to change ourselves. We tell ourselves things like: "It must be me." "If only I tried harder." "It must be because I'm not good enough." "If only I was thinner." Either way the connection is not easily restored.

When we work together (personally or professionally) we mix doing things with sharing information and feelings. We are often made to feel guilty for the amount of time we spend schmoozing or talking about personal things. We are made to feel that we are not getting enough done. Men need to figure out their position in the hierarchy of power before they can get things done. Women first need to develop a cooperative environment among ourselves. We check each other out to determine how safe we feel with one another and how accurately we think we will be judged. We make connections by trying to establish what we have in common with one another. Once we have assessed these connections, then we can get to work.

It is when we begin to form relationships with men that we often come up against a wall of mutual misunderstanding. Deborah Tannen's classic example illustrates the cultural barriers between us:[33]

> Mark and Jennifer are out driving in their car. Mark holds the wheel, Jennifer holds the map.
>
> "I know a shorter way to get there," Mark says, and they proceed to get lost.
>
> "Why don't we stop and ask for directions," Jennifer suggests.

"No," Mark replies, "I know the way." And so they continue.

An hour later Jennifer makes the same suggestion. Mark again refuses. On the third try she demands, "Stop and ask for directions!"

"No," he says with determination, "I'll find it." They continue the trip in tense silence, both unaware of how and why things went wrong.

Mark feels criticized because he doesn't have a cultural context for this experience. He intuitively feels that he knows where he is going. He has a mental picture in his mind, and his sense of spatial relations is better than Jennifer's. He sees Jennifer's advice as criticism, a sign that she thinks he is not capable of figuring things out. According to his logic, if she loved him she'd have confidence in his ability to find the way. He handles his hurt by withdrawing.

Jennifer is unaware of Mark's path-finding skills or of the fact that these skills even exist. She feels hurt and rebuffed when she tries to help Mark with the suggestion that he deal with the situation in the same way that she would by asking for directions. When he doesn't take the advice that she is offering, she interprets his rejection as a sign that he doesn't care for her.

Neither is aware that for Jennifer the way to solve problems is through collaboration, and that for Mark it is to do it alone. For Mark to ask for directions means giving up some power, and thereby ending up feeling inadequate about his abilities. For Jennifer, however, the same act simply involves initiating contact with someone else – an event that might be a potentially positive experience.

Because we have a context for their behavior, we can understand how Mark and Jennifer become locked behind the barriers that these cultural behaviors erect between them. Later on in this book we will use this understanding of gender and development to see how these cultural barriers are recreated in the father-daughter relationship. We will look at how they create conflict in our relationships with girls when we lose ourselves in our formal roles of mother or teacher and begin to communicate in hierarchical fashion like men.

Welcome to Adam's World

The cultural barriers that we encounter in our interpersonal relationships reflect the larger barriers that we experience in the world.
We live in Adam's world, where life is presented to us from a male
perspective and that is assumed to be the norm. It determines the
way we see the world, the way we express ourselves, the kind of language we use, the ideas we consider to be important, and the things
we value. Our institutions are all structured according to this male
point of view. So, too, are most common objects and processes. Take
the computer, for example. How come we all take it for granted that
when it is working it is up and when it is not working it is down?
The male perspective has been the norm for so long that it's difficult for men (and sometimes even for women) to see that perhaps
there is an alternative – another way of being in the world.

Since our society revolves around the male perspective, the
things that men do and the ways that they do them are more highly
valued. The female perspective and the things that women do are
less valued. And because the rules of society are written in male
terms, girls who want to be included in the larger world have to
work harder to find ways of fitting in – often at great expense to
themselves.

The continuum of human behavior in our society is somewhat
lopsided. One of the two cultures is valued more than the other –
and that dominant culture is male. If we lived in a world that
respected the uniqueness of both male and female cultures, we
would each of us be able to move freely back and forth along the
whole continuum of human behavior. Because all men are not the
same and all women are not the same, we could open up a much
wider range of choices for all of us. We could respond to those situations that required a process-oriented approach with skills from
the female culture, and to those where goal-oriented solutions were
more appropriate with responses from the male culture. We could
allow for competitive women and collaborative men in the work-
force. We would value the kind of nurturing that men provide at
home. If we could be bicultural, we could complement one another
and create a much-needed balance in the world.

NOTES

1   Deborah Tannen. *You Just Don't Understand: Women and Men in Conversation*. New York: Ballantine Books, 1990, pp. 49-59, 77, 97-100.

2   J.Z. Rubin, E.J. Provenzano and Z. Luria. "The Eye of the Beholder: Parents' Views on the Sex of Newborns." *American Journal of Orthopsychiatry*, 1974, No. 44, pp. 512-519.

3   C. Smith and B. Lloyd. "Maternal Behavior and Perceived Sex of Infant: Revisited." *Child Development*, 1978, No. 49, pp. 1263-1266.

4   Jeanne H. Block. "Personality Development in Males and Females: The Influence of Differential Socialization." Paper presented as part of the Master Lecture Series at a meeting of the American Psychological Association, New York, September 1979, p. 3.

5   Block.

6   Block.

7   Anne Moir and David Jessel. *Brain Sex: The Real Difference between Men and Women*. New York: Bantam Doubleday Dell, 1991, pp. 33-37.

8   June M. Reinisch. "Fetal Hormones, the Brain and Human Sex Differences: A Heuristic Integrative Review of the Recent Literature." *Archives of Sexual Behavior*, 1974, No. 3, pp. 51-90.

9   Moir and Jessel.

10 Deborah Blum. *Sex on the Brain: The Biological Differences between Men and Women*. New York: Viking, 1997.

11 Moir and Jessel.

12 Michael Hutchison. *The Anatomy of Sex and Power: An Investigation of Mind-Body Politics*. New York: William Morrow, 1990, p. 168.

13 Joanne Berger-Sweeney. "The Developing Brain: Genes, Environment and Behavior." AAAS Symposium, February 9, 1996.

14 Sigmund Freud. *A General Introduction to Psychoanalysis*. J. Riviere, trans. New York: Permabooks, 1953.

15 Erik Erikson. *Identity, Youth and Crisis*. New York: W.W. Norton, 1968.

16 Janet L. Surrey. "The Self-in-Relation: A Theory of Women's Development" in Judith Jordon, Alexandra G. Kaplan, Jean Baker Miller, Irene P. Stiver and Janet L. Surrey. *Women's Growth in Connection: Writings from the Stone Center*. New York: Guilford Press, 1991, pp. 51-64.

17 Surrey.

18 Carol Gilligan and Lyn Mikel Brown. *Meeting at the Crossroads: Women's Psychology and Girls' Development*. Cambridge: Harvard University Press, 1992.

19 Surrey.

20 Surrey.

21 Surrey.

22 B. Schieffelin and E. Ochs. *Language Socialization across Cultures*. New York: Cambridge University Press, 1986, p. 2.

23 B. Whiting and C. Edwards. *Children of Different Worlds*. Cambridge: Harvard University Press, 1988.

24 Tannen.

25 Tannen.

26 Tannen.

27 Tannen.

28 Amy Sheldon. "Pickle Fights: Gendered Talk in Preschool Disputes" in Deborah Tannen, ed. *Gender and Conversational Interaction*. New York: Oxford University Press, 1993, pp. 83-109.

29 Sheldon.

30 Deborah Tannen. "He Said, She Said." PBS, 1994.

31 Tannen.

32 Tannen.

33 Tannen.

2

Growing Up Female

Whenever I go to speak or do workshops with groups of girls or women, I guide them through a fantasy, taking them back to the time before puberty – when they were eight years old. I invite my audience to share their insights about the changes that they see in themselves now. Many of us remember being eight as a time of much greater freedom. We didn't have to please everyone then or worry about how we looked. Despite the fact that we have more choices now, eight was a time when we were not so burdened by responsibilities in our lives. According to psychologist Emily Hancock, most of us recognize the age of eight as the transitional point in childhood between fully knowing who we are and beginning to lose touch with ourselves.[1]

In the period between preschool and puberty, girls manage life better than boys. They mature faster. Their female brain structure equips them to learn math and reading skills earlier. They develop better control of their small motor skills, which facilitates their handwriting.[2] Until girls begin puberty, they generally feel good about themselves and about their abilities. They are most creative, most assertive and most in tune with themselves and with the world around them.[3] At eight years of age, girls are physically equal to boys. They weigh the same and are just as tall. They can run as fast, jump as high and hit a ball just as well as boys.

As they proceed through middle childhood, girls acquire skills in logic and strategy that allow them to problem-solve and to cope with many of the ordinary things in life. Until the ages of eleven and twelve, they are also psychologically healthier and have fewer behavioral problems than boys.[4] At least they are if they have not been sexually abused or been victims of violence.

Before girls reach adolescence, they can be quite self-sufficient. They can choose their own clothes, fix a leaky faucet, bake a cake and decide how to spend their free time. They have the cognitive ability to reason and to figure things out. Their capacity for memory is greater than it has ever been before.[5]

At this stage in their development, friends become very important to girls. Girls spend a good deal of energy learning and practicing the intricacies of relationships, and in absorbing the rules of their peer groups. They now have the cognitive ability to recognize that other people have feelings, needs and reasons for acting as they do. They are able to see things from another person's perspective and understand another person's point of view. These friendships influence the kinds of clothes girls wear, the activities that interest them, and the things they do.

Until girls reach adolescence, they are able to have open and honest relationships with others. They actively and unselfconsciously fight with one another with passion and spontaneity – because they have confidence in their ability to settle their differences and make up. They know that feeling jealous and angry (and even being mean) are part of what happens in relationships, and that fighting and making up are the elements that build trust. They trust their belief in fairness. They are sure that the rift in the relationship will be repaired if only they can make the other person see things through their point of view. But as girls approach adolescence, they reach an impasse in their psychological growth and development.[6]

When twelve-year-old girls enter seventh grade, they have an edge on boys. When they leave, this is reversed. In this period between childhood and adulthood, girls' bodies begin to change and this alters their lives as well. They begin to suffer from depression, stress and other signs of psychological distress. They begin to worry a lot about their safety and the safety of others, about the unknown and especially about the way that they look.[7] The transition into adolescence may be difficult for all children, but girls' self-esteem drops further than boys' and never catches up. The greatest drop occurs in the period between elementary school and junior high.[8]

As their hormones trigger changes in their bodies at the onset of puberty, society (in the form of parents, teachers, the media and other institutions) begins to prepare them for other changes in their lives. Girls are required to make major adaptations in how they see themselves and how they interact with the world. They experience major changes in the way they carry on their relationships. They embrace the societal image of the perfect girl and in the process begin to discount the things they value most about themselves. They start to live their lives in translation, in order to fit into and be included by the male-defined world. Many begin to learn the language of fat.

Developing a False Self

Carol Gilligan and Lyn Mikel Brown researched the psychological development of young women over a period of five years. They studied 100 girls between the ages of seven and eighteen years at Laurel School for girls in Cleveland, Ohio, between 1986 and 1990. Because girls develop their identity or sense of self in the context of their relationships, as chapter 1 pointed out, they measured the changes in girls' sense of self by studying the changes in their relationships as they grew up. Once a year over the course of the study, approximately 25 girls in the first, fourth, seventh and tenth grades were given the same series of questions. These encouraged the girls to talk with the researchers about their thoughts and feelings about themselves and about their relationships.[9]

Eight- and nine-year-old girls in the study spoke about their lives with authority. They were sure of themselves and were very definite in their opinions and feelings. They began their sentences with "I feel ..." "I know ..." They made it very clear they were most definitely the center of their own experiences and challenged anyone who told them what to think.[10] Gilligan and Brown found that girls will flourish if they are allowed to be truthful about their feelings and opinions, and if the people in their lives engage with them honestly.

Gilligan and Brown point out a fundamental paradox that develops in girls' lives. On one hand, the desire for connection and mutually responsive and engaging relationships makes up an integral part of female identity. Yet when girls become adolescents, they learn to silence themselves in their relationships rather than risk open conflict that might lead to rejection, isolation and perhaps violence against themselves.[11]

During puberty, girls fall victim to the "tyranny of kind and nice."[12] They are bombarded with messages from all around them that it is better to be polite and not hurt anyone's feelings than to be honest and say what they really think and feel. In order to relate in a way that is socially acceptable, girls develop a phony or "polite" voice and lie about what they see happening around them. Where honesty once was the glue that held their relationships together, girls are now taught that it is a weapon that will drive their relationships apart. Early adolescence becomes a confusing time for them.

As adults, most of us have a lot of practice being kind and nice. We all cultivate in various degrees a phony or polite voice that has become integrated into who we are. It's the voice that we use in public when we are afraid of saying what we really think. It's the one that we use when someone drops in unannounced and we assure them that they are not imposing – we even offer them coffee – while deep inside, we hope they will soon leave. It's our response when we sit through endless phone conversations with clenched teeth because we are afraid to hurt the other person by telling them that we have other things to do and would really just like to get off the phone.

Girls make further changes in how they relate to others when they become interested in boys. They must now accommodate themselves to people of a different gender who do not have the same social skills or place the same degree of importance on relationships that they do. In order to adapt to the superficial and idealized kinds of relationships that are required of them, girls suppress additional parts of themselves. They learn that taking care of the emotional needs of others means setting aside their own feelings and perceptions.

In the process of learning to relate as adults, girls move back and forth across a chasm between what is expected of them and what they know to be true. They know deep down in their hearts that what they value most is their honesty and directness and their commitment to standing up for what they believe. At the same time, they look around and see that the popular girls are the ones that are nice and fit in. Popular girls deal with their conflicts by shopping and never ever challenge the status quo.

Girls struggle with a terrible choice: they can remain who they are – and thus be different from their friends and risk losing them – or they can become like everyone else. In the process of trying to conform, they begin to misplace pieces of themselves. According to Mary Pipher, author of *Reviving Ophelia*, girls split into two selves in order to be accepted socially.[13] The real self is like an inner self that contains all the thoughts and feelings that society tells them they cannot express – such as anger, jealousy and sexuality. The false self is an outer shell that they create to reflect back the qualities and responses society expects from them.

Girls at twelve and thirteen years are still able to distinguish the difference between their real self and their false one. After thirteen, they are struggling just to retain their inner self. In the groups that I have facilitated, the most pressing issues concerned relationships with parents and friends. Over and over again, the girls dealt with the profound question that all women struggle with: "How do I have a relationship with you and still be me, if I always have to worry about hurting you?"

As they get older, they slowly succumb to the pressures being exerted on them by society. Thirteen-year-old girls no longer confidently respond with "I." Instead, they cautiously say, "I don't know" or "whatever." Though their real self peeps out every now and again, for the most part they have already begun to hold back what they think and feel.

The more practiced girls become at using their false self and accommodating themselves to other peoples' needs, the harder it is for them to tell the difference between what they feel and think inside and what they project outside. Soon the false self becomes the only one they know. At fifteen, girls answer questions with a shrug and "you know." The source of their information is now outside themselves.[14]

As their real self becomes buried and the false one takes its place, girls begin to dissociate themselves from their experiences, from their feelings and from themselves. They lose their voice – the confidence to speak out and state their opinions – as well as their ability to take their experiences seriously. They stop being the center of their own experiences and become hostage to the ever-changing opinions of others. As they look outside for self-definition, many find it in the numbers on the scale.

Becoming Barbie: The Perfect Girl

As girls approach adolescence, they discover that the very skills that empowered them as girls now betray them as they become women and are judged from a male perspective. Because male culture is based on competition and detachment, those qualities that make girls unique are reframed so that being female now means being needy, dependent, hysterical and having trouble making up your mind. It means always needing approval and never getting things done. Girls constantly receive conflicting messages about what they value and know to be true about themselves, and what society expects from them. First and foremost, girls are expected to attain the kind of beauty that is physically impossible for most to achieve. They are rewarded for being passive, for exhibiting self-control and for putting the needs of others ahead of themselves. At the same time, they must nurture the very qualities that we associate predominately with being male. To succeed in the larger world, they must be independent, competitive, aggressive and goal-oriented.

Whenever I ask girls or women to share their images of the perfect person – regardless of their own race and ethnicity – they are almost always unanimous in their list. The perfect girl is Barbie. She is tall, thin, blonde, white, beautiful, competent, confident, independent, young, athletic, sexy and powerful. She has big white teeth, big lips and big breasts. She makes a lot of money and doesn't need anybody else. She is always in control and never has PMS or zits.

When I ask girls what they value about being a girl, they list friends, family, boys, pets, bubble baths, boys, reading books, playing sports, hanging out and boys. (Later on as adults they will add children, partners, families, friends, security, home, feeling good about themselves and liking the kind of work that they do.) When I ask girls to name the things that they like about each other, it's difficult for them to see beyond pretty and nice.

The model of perfection that is held out to girls is one-dimensional. It doesn't account for the sheer messiness, the ups and downs and the insecurities and stresses of real life. Because this model is unattainable, girls always end up feeling as if there is something wrong with them, no matter how hard they try. Because none of the things that girls value, and none of the qualities that make up the real female culture are reflected back to them positively by society, girls soon learn to devalue themselves.

Living Our Lives in Translation

Because we live in Adam's world, girls must translate their thoughts and experiences from a female-oriented language and style to the male-oriented one if they want to fit in. This means that girls learn to live their lives in translation in order to accommodate themselves to Adam's rules. Let's see how this happens.

Imagine that you are having coffee with a small group of women. They could be your friends or they could be colleagues at work. You're talking about a book you read, a movie you saw or a situation that happened in your life. The discussion is very lively and animated. You all have different points of view and you all want to share your opinions. A man walks into the room, and then another. What happens to the discussion? Most likely it dies. The conversation becomes less spontaneous and you become more self-conscious. The focus shifts to the men, who take over its direction and set a different tone for the discussion. Later on, you are asked to present your opinions on the same book, movie or situation to a large group in a meeting. As you consider how you might phrase things for this mixed audience, it's quite possible that you wonder if your opinions are at all important and begin to question whether indeed you have anything at all to say.

Like anybody who must constantly translate from one language to another, girls lose most of their nuances, context and frames of reference when they express themselves in male terms. Soon they begin to qualify their opinions with phrases such as "This is probably wrong, but ..." This makes them feel trivialized, so they start to trivialize themselves. They begin their sentences with "I'm sorry to bother you, but ..." They soon cease to speak, because they feel unheard. They withhold their opinions because they feel they have nothing important to say. They gradually lose their ability to know what they really think, because they are afraid of being laughed at or being considered wrong. They question the validity of their own experiences, discount their own abilities and continue the process of dissociating from themselves.

Learning the Language of Fat

Girls approaching puberty are encouraged to repress their feelings, which stops them talking about the important issues in their lives. As they try to fit into the male culture, they lose their sense of identity and devalue the very qualities and characteristics that make them unique. These feelings don't just go away. Many girls associate the societal restrictions that are imposed upon them with the inevitable weight gain and increase in body fat that occur during puberty. They try to deal with the new restrictions in their lives by focusing on these changes in their bodies. They focus on their reflected external image instead of on their real internal selves. Girls deflect their feelings back onto their bodies and encode them in the language of fat.

 ## Time Out for Yourself

- **Look back in time**. Think back to when you were eight.
    - What did you like doing?
    - Who were your friends?
    - What did you look forward to?
    - How did you feel about yourself?
    - Remember back to a decision that you made at that time – a decision that you knew was right with every fiber of your being. Remember what that felt like and try to hold on to that feeling. Now think about your present life and how you feel about yourself.
    - How is life different for you now that you are older?
    - What changes have taken place in the way that you feel about yourself?
    - Can you pinpoint when these changes started to happen?

- **Pay attention to your phony voice**.[15] Sit down with a cup of coffee or tea at the end of the day. Think about the people you interacted with. As you think about each specific situation, ask yourself if you said what you really wanted to say. If you didn't, ask yourself what you would have said if you didn't have to worry about hurting somebody else's feelings or losing your job. Say the words out loud just to make them real.

- **Examine your myths of perfection**. Imagine that you were a perfect person. What would you look like? What would you be doing in your life? What qualities would you possess? How would your life be different than it is now? Make a list of what's important to you. How is this list different from your idea of the perfect person? What would you give up to attain your image of perfection?

NOTES

1 Emily Hancock. *The Girl Within*. New York: Ballantine Books, 1989, p. 9.
2 C. Shakeshaft. "A Gender at Risk." *Phi Delta Kappan*, March 1986, Vol. 67, No. 7, pp. 500-503.
3 Hancock.
4 D. Offord, M.H. Boyle, P. Szatmari, et al. "Ontario Child and Health Study II: Six Month Prevalence of Disorder and Rates of Service Utilization." *Archives of General Psychiatry*, 1987, Vol. 44, pp. 832-836.
5 Laurence Steinberg and Jay Belsky. *Infancy, Childhood & Adolescence: Development in Context*. New York: McGraw Hill, 1991, p. 344.
6 Carol Gilligan and Lyn Mikel Brown. *Meeting at the Crossroads: Women's Psychology and Girls' Development*. Cambridge: Harvard University Press, 1992.
7 Offord, et al.
8 American Association of University Women Educational Foundation. *Shortchanging Girls, Shortchanging America*. Washington, DC, 1990, p. 17.
9 Gilligan and Brown.
10 Gilligan and Brown.
11 Gilligan and Brown.
12 Gilligan and Brown.
13 Mary Pipher. *Reviving Ophelia: Saving the Selves of Adolescent Girls*. New York: Ballantine Books, 1994, pp. 19-23.
14 Catherine Steiner-Adair spoke of these changes in 1995, at a conference in Toronto sponsored by the National Eating Disorder Information Centre and the Toronto General Hospital.
15 Catherine Steiner-Adair gave a wonderful illustration of girls' phony voices in 1995 at a conference in Toronto.

BUILDING
OUR SKILLS

■

*Decoding the
Language of Fat*

3

When Girls Feel Fat

It's almost impossible for us to grow up female without worrying about our weight, without developing ambivalent feelings about food, without ever apologizing for eating. Even though we have been told time and time again that being overweight is not necessarily unhealthy and that diets don't work, it's hard not to be seduced by the relentless message that everyone should want to be thin. We are bombarded with the idea that we can change our body shape if only we try hard enough. We are coerced into thinking that there is something wrong with us if we choose to accept the body we have.

When I was growing up, my mother and all her friends dieted in an attempt to "improve" their figures. By the age of fifteen, I was following in her footsteps and desperately trying to change my shape. Today, six- and seven-year-old girls are concerned about their weight. Standing at the cusp of puberty, nine-year-old girls talk about feeling fat before their bodies have even begun to change. At ten and eleven, feeling fat has been incorporated into their everyday language. It influences how they see themselves and the way they interact with the world.

As girls enter puberty, more than half of them will tell you that they feel better if they are on a diet because it gives them a feeling of being in control of themselves. By the time they reach high school, many girls will already be using laxatives, diuretics, appetite suppressants, vomiting, fasting and excessive exercise as means of coping with the changes in their bodies and in their lives.

It's hardly surprising then that when girls start to talk about feeling fat, we adults get really scared. When feeling fat becomes a consistent theme in their talk, we begin to worry about eating disorders. And no wonder! In the past fifteen years, school nurses have begun to see ever-increasing numbers of elementary school girls with anorexia nervosa. Nurses in high schools express real concern about the number of girls they see who binge and purge.

While most girls worry about their weight, not everybody tries to control their weight to the same extent. Many girls may experiment with some of the behaviors, but not everybody develops an eating disorder. Nor do eating disorders develop overnight. Yet feeling fat exacts a high price from girls even if it doesn't ultimately end in their getting sick. Feeling fat and worrying about weight affects how girls feel about themselves. It affects their relationships with other people, their self-confidence and their sense of their own abilities.

When girls focus on their external image at the expense of their internal selves, when they worry constantly about weight and feeling fat, they disconnect from their feelings and their bodies. Girls come to see taking care of themselves in terms of looking good. They become overly concerned with other people's opinions, especially those of their friends. The need to please other people makes it difficult for them to make healthy choices and to say no – to smoking, to unprotected sex and to getting into a car with a drunk driver – even when they know they are putting themselves at risk.

Why Girls Feel Fat

To help girls understand why they feel fat, we need to know what this means to them. We need to know the relationship between feeling fat and getting sick. We need a context for how eating disorders develop and what they actually mean.

Part of the definition of growing up female means that at some point you will feel fat. We've all felt fat. We've all had days when we've weighed ourselves in the morning and felt crushed when the numbers seemed to climb. We've all gone on diets when things around us were stressful, thinking that if we couldn't control our lives, maybe we could control our weight.

Most of us are quite familiar with feeling fat. It seems so normal to us that it's hard to accept that feeling fat isn't really a feeling at all and that it is unrelated to body weight. Fat people feel fat. Thin people feel fat. Yet nobody feels fat all the time. Let's say that at one o'clock you feel perfectly fine, and then at ten past one you feel fat. It is unlikely that you have swallowed a watermelon! Rather, you have encoded the stressful or negative feelings you are experiencing at a particular time into a language of fat and self-deprecation. Let's see how that works:

Stacey stands in front of her closet holding up a pair of jeans. "I'm not going to school today," she wails, "I'm so fat!"

"No, you're not," responds her mother Gina.

"Yes, I am," yells Stacey, grabbing a red T-shirt and throwing it on the floor.

"No, you're not," says Gina, trying her best to help.

"Yes, I am! Just look at the size of my thighs!"

"Your thighs look fine," responds Gina, in an attempt to make things better. "Why don't you wear your blue skirt? It's your favorite and it really looks good on you."

"My thighs are so fat. I'm so fat," insists Stacey, as the skirt joins the pile of clothes on the floor.

"You're not fat."

"Yes, I am!"

"No, you're not!"

"You just don't understand," yells Stacey, as she storms angrily out of the room.

Stacey's dad, Kevin, hears the commotion and comes rushing into the hall. "What's going on?" he asks.

"Stacey doesn't want to go to school because she feels fat. I keep telling her that she's not fat and that her blue skirt really looks good on her," says Gina.

"Well," Kevin says to Stacey, "If you stopped snacking after school, you probably wouldn't feel so fat."

"I knew it," cries Stacey as she runs out of the house, "I knew you thought I was fat."

Clare buries her face in the pillow and laments with despair, "Michael doesn't want to be my boyfriend – I know it's because I'm fat."

"You're not fat," says her friend Megan as she tries to console her, "and anyway, Michael is a dweeb."

"I am fat," cries Clare, "and I'll never have a boyfriend. Nobody will want me because I'm so fat."

"No, you're not," insists Megan.

"Yes, I am!"

"No, you're not," exclaims Megan in frustration, knowing how it feels to feel fat but not knowing what else to do or say to help her friend.

If these sound familiar, it's because we've probably all played them out hundreds and hundreds of times. We've been the ones who have felt fat and nothing anybody could say would make the feelings go away. We've also been on the flip side of this dialogue and felt as if we were hitting our head against a brick wall trying to help someone else cope with feeling fat.

In these scenarios that I've described, Stacey may be reluctant to go to school because she has a test that is making her anxious or because the boy who sits behind her harasses her every chance he gets, or because her best friend is ignoring her and she is feeling hurt. When Clare is able to express her disappointment that Michael doesn't want to be her boyfriend, she opens the door for Megan to share her own insecurities over boys.

Most of us know of only two responses when girls feel fat. We can either disagree with them – in which case they don't believe us

– or we can agree with them, and then they get angry and won't speak to us further. Most of the time we try to make it better or tell them what to do, because that's how we've been taught. It's also what we think they want. But no matter how hard we try to talk them out of it, we are usually met with resistance because feeling fat is not really a feeling. It is a *code*.

The Language of Fat

When I first started my work as a therapist and began developing workshops for women who were preoccupied with their weight, I was invited to appear on a radio call-in show. At first I was very excited. I was going to be a big shot – local woman makes good! The euphoria lasted until the morning of the radio show.

When I woke up that morning all I could feel was fat. I kept on telling myself that if only I were thinner, the radio show would be a greater success. Doesn't make sense, does it?

Once I became aware of what I was doing, I got curious about what was underneath this "feeling." I realized that I was scared. What if the show began and I couldn't even speak properly? What if I made some kind of mistake? What if someone called in and I didn't know the right answer? My mother would be listening and so would her friends, and so would my relatives, and so would all my friends. When I finally decoded the message underneath the language of fat, I was able to express my feelings of anxiety and deal with those fears. I was still a bit nervous when I arrived at the radio station, but I was able to do the show because I had acknowledged and addressed what was really going on.

We've been taught that it's not all right for us to express certain feelings. We've been encouraged to keep certain opinions to ourselves. It may be because we don't know what these are, or because it is just not safe to show them, or because we think they are wrong. We get angry with ourselves (or don't like ourselves or don't like our bodies) when we don't have any other way of directly expressing our feelings. We turn our feelings and experiences against ourselves and put ourselves down.

The fabric of everyday life is made up of many small events that are interwoven with a multitude of feelings. Yet ask any woman how her day was and she is most likely to answer "fine." Ask her what happened that day and unless she was hit by a bus or a major disaster occurred, she is most likely to say "nothing." We've learned to transform our self-expression into self-repression and to redirect our feelings against ourselves.

A friend of mine used to tell the story of the couple whose car door was stuck. The man asked: "What's wrong with the door? It won't open." The woman asked: "What's wrong with me? I can't open the door." Where men have been socialized to handle distress by striking out, we have been socialized to blame ourselves. We say: "I'm so mad at myself," or "I just hate myself." This carries over to our bodies when we say: "I hate my stomach," or "I hate my thighs," or "I feel so fat."

Instead of expressing things directly, we encode our feelings and experiences in the language of fat. We feel fat when we're angry and we feel fat when we're sad. We feel fat when we are disappointed or when we feel lonely or jealous or are sexually frustrated or even sexually aroused. Because it's hard for us to express even the feelings that we consider to be the good ones, sometimes we even feel fat when we're happy and things are going well in our lives.

Because our society considers fat bad, every time we feel fat, what we are saying is "I don't like my body" – which really means "I don't like myself the way I am." We have to remember that this is *learned behavior*.

Some of us feel fat only occasionally and some of us feel fat a lot. Sometimes we encode so many of our feelings and experiences in the language of fat that it seems as if it is the only language that we speak. We become so preoccupied with what feeling fat means to us that we fail to address the issues that lie underneath. As the real feelings become more intense, the code becomes more difficult to decipher. We first try to deal with our discomfort by dieting. Because that doesn't help us decipher the code and express what we feel underneath, we soon begin to feel even worse. And so we up the ante by breaking the diet (only to repeat the cycle all over again) or by beginning to purge and fast.

Understanding the Continuum

When I started out in private practice in 1980, bingeing, purging and fasting were so uncommon that girls and women engaging in these behaviors were considered to have an established eating disorder. Today, these behaviors are so much a part of the normal teen culture that whenever we talk to high school students about eating disorders, many of them have a hard time applying the information to themselves. They just worry about their weight. It's other girls that take it too far and who are at risk.

Sometimes girls will experiment with the behaviors that we associate with eating disorders and stop without any kind of intervention or counseling. They either resolve the contentious issues in their lives or find other ways of dealing with them. Some girls do get caught up in a preoccupation with food and weight. As this preoccupation and the behaviors associated with it intensify, some of these girls eventually develop an eating disorder.

Eating disorders and the preoccupation with food and weight exist along a continuum, which is a line that illustrates how things progress. Sometimes it shows progression in stages. Sometimes it shows increasing quantity or intensity, where you begin with a little and end up with a lot. The continuum of food and weight preoccupation shows the stages that occur between the time when girls feel fat and when they end up in the hospital with dangerously low weight. Let's follow the continuum and see how this works.

Imagine the girls in your local school:

- A very large number of the girls will start to feel fat by the end of sixth grade – and most certainly in seventh grade. Many of them will tell you that their mothers worry about their own weight.

- Many of these girls will become preoccupied with food and weight. They will think a lot about what they eat, and feel fat quite often.

- A fair number of these girls will experiment with dieting, bingeing, purging and exercising to excess by the time they are in high school.

- Some girls will get caught up in these dynamics and might develop eating disorders.
- A small number of these girls will develop medical complications from the behaviors.
- A few will finally end up in the hospital at real medical risk.

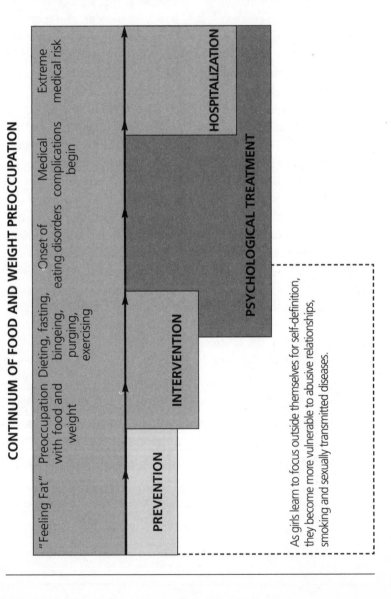

CONTINUUM OF FOOD AND WEIGHT PREOCCUPATION

"Feeling Fat" | Preoccupation with food and weight | Dieting, fasting, bingeing, purging, exercising | Onset of eating disorders | Medical complications begin | Extreme medical risk

PREVENTION

INTERVENTION

PSYCHOLOGICAL TREATMENT

HOSPITALIZATION

As girls learn to focus outside themselves for self-definition, they become more vulnerable to abusive relationships, smoking and sexually transmitted diseases.

Developing an Eating Disorder

While many girls feel fat, not all girls will develop an eating disorder. Anorexia and bulimia are part of a continuum of disordered eating that includes compulsive eating, chronic "normalized" dieting, weight preoccupation and body dissatisfaction. An eating disorder develops when the behaviors around food and weight preoccupation escalate – when they become such an obsession that everything girls do, and all of their feelings, are determined by what they have or haven't eaten that day and by the numbers on the bathroom scale.

While eating disorders are expressions of food/weight issues, they are not merely problems with food, or with weight, and have very little to do with physiological hunger. In fact, most girls with eating disorders can't even tell when they are hungry. For girls with eating disorders, food in itself is not the issue. Food does not cause eating disorders. However, an erratic relationship with food helps fuel these behaviors once they begin.

Food is the focus for behaviors that are triggered primarily by psychological need. Girls use food and the preoccupation with weight to deal with feelings that are too painful or are considered inappropriate to express – such as loneliness, insecurity, anger, sexuality and need. They use it to deal with tension and anxiety, with emotional conflict, and with difficulties that they cannot express or resolve. In adolescence, girls use food and weight as a means of dealing with their transition into an adult world that devalues the relational structure of the female culture and undervalues the ways in which they interact with the world.

For the compulsive overeater and for the bulimic who does not vomit, food is a way of stuffing down or anesthetizing these feelings. For the bulimic who does vomit, food provides the means to symbolically discharge the feelings through the purging. For the anorexic, not eating provides symbolic control.

We all have a need to feel in control, to have a certain amount of order and certainty in our lives. To feel in control is to feel one's own power to make choices, to say yes or no. Imagine what it would be like, for example, to go through an entire week when you could never say no. Every time someone wanted something from you, or you felt that they did, you had to say yes. Think about how powerless you would feel if you could never have any boundaries in your life because you were afraid of hurting someone else. When girls feel they don't have this right, when taking control of their own lives means facing what to them means rejection and isolation, they create a sense of control that seems less threatening to them. We've all learned that although you can't always control your life, you can control what you eat.

Eating disorder behaviors externalize the parts of girls that are not acceptable to them or to society. Because the perfect woman is thin, passive, independent, unemotional and in control, girls dissociate from those parts of themselves that do not fit this image. They redirect the imperfect parts of themselves onto their fat, their bulimia, their anorexia – as if these were separate entities with lives of their own, containing all the feelings that are too scary to acknowledge or too difficult to express.

Girls develop eating disorders for a multitude of reasons. There is no one factor. The underlying causes are as complicated and as different as are the girls themselves. Girls who mature early weigh more than their peers. Early dieting behavior changes their metabolism so that they have to engage in more and more risk-taking activities in order to lose weight. Girls who have a tendency toward perfectionism, who have low self-esteem, who have a sense of ineffectiveness in their lives, who lack intimate connections and/or who have experienced changes or losses in their major relationships are often at greater risk. So are girls who have been sexually or physically abused, experienced a recent divorce in the family, or whose parents are chronically depressed or abuse alcohol or drugs. Ineffective communication in families, rigid boundaries that don't give girls room to grow, or a lack of boundaries that makes them feel unsafe are also contributing factors. Girls who are teased about their weight are also at risk as well as those who live in a culture of dieting – where their mothers and friends diet and where they read teen magazines that reinforce a "thin" image.

Eating disorders can occur at different developmental stages.

The most common time of onset is adolescence, when girls' bodies and lives begin to change in dramatic fashion. Most girls go on diets at the most stressful times in their lives. Involvement in intensive activities that emphasize a specific body shape or thinness (i.e., dancing and competitive sports) also tend to put young girls at risk.

Underlying all these factors are the adaptations that girls must make as they grow up female in a male-defined world. Underlying all the personal reasons why girls feel fat are the societal pressures to be thin and beautiful, combined with the general psychological distress that comes from growing up female in a male-defined world.

As you can see from the continuum, two people talking to each other about eating disorders can easily have two totally different pictures in their mind. When girls and women are at the beginning of the continuum, it's more appropriate to see their behavior as a psychological means of coping with the world.

But when girls and women reach the extreme end of the continuum where they are finally at medical risk, eating disorders are addressed from a medical perspective. Because there are such different beliefs about the nature of eating disorders and the preoccupation with food and weight, it is important for you to come to your own understanding. What you believe will influence how you deal with a girl who feels fat, and how she will come to perceive herself.

You may want to know more about eating disorders or may be worried that someone you love is at risk. At the end of this book in the Resources section, I have provided suggestions for books to read and listed organizations in the United States and Canada that you can contact to find out what is available in your area.

4

Getting to What's Underneath

If we are going to prevent eating disorders and help girls avoid the emotional, psychological and physical entrapment of the preoccupation with food and weight, we must turn our attention to the beginning of the continuum – just at the point where girls begin to feel fat. Because feelings don't go away even if we want them to, we can only begin to help girls address what lies beneath the surface when we can help them identify their real concerns.

The Just for Girls Program

In 1992, I developed the *Just for Girls* program, intending to help girls "safely navigate the rocky road through adolescence and avoid pitfalls such as eating disorders and the preoccupation with food and weight." (*Just for Girls* was originally developed as the *Girls in the 90s* program. The name was changed to honor the new millennium.)

I envisioned prevention as a way of intervening with high school girls who were already experimenting with bingeing, purging and dieting. I would facilitate each group with a public health nurse, school nurse or counselor that I trained for this work. My co-facil-itator would in turn train other nurses or counselors. But things didn't work out quite that way.

My ideas received a lot of support from professionals and other adults in the community. Everyone saw the need for such a pro-gram, except the girls that we were trying to reach. The girls who participated in our initial sessions acknowledged that they all wor-ried about their weight – but felt that this was normal. They all knew about eating disorders, but felt that this information didn't apply to them. While each and every one of them supported the idea of a group and knew others who would benefit, nobody both-ered to come.

We then lowered the age group of our target population to those in grades eight and nine, and modified what we said in an effort to reach girls who hadn't even begun to experiment with diets. We took the emphasis off eating disorders and just talked about *feeling fat*. We went into the schools to show films and talk about groups. Girls were enthusiastic. Almost all of them felt fat. They liked the idea of a group – what appealed to them most was the idea of a place and time to just hang out and talk. But once again no one would commit to participating in a program that did not address their more immediate concerns. What if they came to the group but didn't want to talk about their weight all the time? What if they just wanted to talk about relationships?

Finally, a trio of seventh grade girls was brought to a group by their mothers. They returned the next session with their sixth grade friends and gave us an earful of advice. They acknowledged times when they felt fat, ugly or stupid and were more than willing to tell us what lay underneath. But then they said: "Don't just talk about food or weight or body image, because it's not just about that. It's about what else we do and what we want – all the things that concern us."

And so we altered the program. Now the *Just for Girls* program looks at everything that happens to girls in the process of growing up female that encourages them to lose their sense of themselves and to begin defining themselves through the numbers on a scale.

It focuses on healthy development and on helping girls maintain their voice. It puts into practice the information about gender and female development and eating disorders that I've set forth here in the earlier chapters.

The program teaches girls to recognize and decode the language of fat before it becomes integrated into the ways in which they interpret and respond to situations in their lives, and before it becomes a major substitution for their feelings.

Just for Girls is structured as an open discussion group. The girls involved insisted on the word *open* because it meant that they could feel free to talk about any issues. It is set right at the beginning of the continuum, so *Just for Girls* has little direct connection with eating disorders. It has more to do with the experiences of girls as they go through puberty and attempt to become women in a world designed for men.

While it's important for girls to be able to express themselves, girls also need to know that they have a right to the way they think and feel. They need to know that they are not weird or different or wrong. The *Just for Girls* group leaders validate the girls' stories and the ways in which they tell them. They provide girls with an understanding of their concerns, experiences and feelings that is framed in the context of female development and socialization. At a time when girls are at risk of losing their culture, this helps them celebrate their interdependence with the relevant people in their lives and highlights the importance to them of those relationships. The adults also provide girls with an understanding of the societal pressures that they face – so that they are able to understand why they feel the way they do.

While certain groups are centered mainly on discussion, some facilitators use role-playing, journal writing, drawing and various other activities to encourage girls to explore their stories and express their concerns. Girls are encouraged to experiment by developing different endings for their stories to make them feel better about themselves. This gives them an opportunity to try out new behavior and practice their communication skills. The group process allows girls to learn how to support each other and to recognize that they are not alone in what they feel.

Each group runs for a period of ten to twelve weeks after school hours, and sometimes in a safe venue away from the school grounds. During discussions, the girls use a "talking stick," a custom adapted from the North American Indians. The talking stick is passed around the circle. Only the person currently holding it may speak, for as long as she pleases without being interrupted. The use of the talking stick ensures that each girl has a chance to articulate her own concerns and be listened to. This reinforces within the group that what she has to say is important and provides her with an opportunity to develop her voice and retain her self-confidence.

Talking about the Grungies: Decoding the Language of Fat

Just for Girls helps girls to recognize *grungies* – a term that we coined to describe the situation when girls feel fat, ugly or stupid. Talking about the grungies teaches girls to recognize all the other aspects of their negative voice. Once girls come to recognize their grungies, they learn to decode them, to tell the stories about their real concerns, and then express the feelings that lie underneath.

Eleven-year-old Lindsay begins to talk about her grungie in her grade six group. "I felt fat on Sunday," she begins. When we ask her what was going on at that time she says, "We had our spring performance for my jazz dancing class. I was in the front row and I felt fat." From further exploration we find that Lindsay was wearing a two-piece outfit. She felt self-conscious and uncomfortable because people were looking at her developing body. We help Lindsay identify her feelings and we agree that it's no wonder that she felt the way that she did. We let her know that other girls in the same situation feel the same way. We talk about how girls are "supposed to feel proud" when people make comments about their bodies, when what they really feel is bad.

In the grade seven group, twelve-year-old Cara talks about feeling stupid. It happened when the teacher asked her a question in class. She says that if she didn't feel stupid she might feel a bit angry. "Mr. Smith always calls on me when he knows I don't know the answer," she tells us. "It's just not fair." The other girls then begin to air similar grievances. We role-play what they might really want to say.

Thirteen-year-old Kate felt fat when she went swimming. It happened when she saw other eighth grade girls begin to whisper among themselves. "I knew that they were talking about me," she said. "I hate when people talk about me behind my back." Kate's grungie opens the door to a discussion about the dark side of friendship – about secrets and cliques and the pain of being excluded when your best friend finds somebody else.

Meeting the Girls in the Groups

While girls in the various groups had many issues in common, the differing degrees of importance that they placed on these issues and their insights into their own behavior reflected their different stages of female development. Later in this book you will hear the individual voices as they talk about their concerns. In this chapter, I've created a composite of the various groups so that you can enter into the world of these girls and get a glimpse into their lives. This may help provide you with an understanding of what it is like today to be ten, eleven, twelve and thirteen and of what's underneath the grungies when girls feel fat.

SIXTH GRADE GIRLS

Sixth grade girls were always giggly and had difficulty sitting still. They came to the group because they could talk about anything and because it was fun. The girls loved to role-play and to act out situations. They loved to draw. We always did some kind of physical activity to help them discharge the pent-up energy they brought with them. We provided the girls in each group with journals and encouraged them to write about the stories underneath their grungies. In one group, the girls created an advice column. In another, one of the girls wrote a book and shared the chapters as she went along.

As preteens, girls in sixth grade often felt unheard. They were the "forgotten" group, falling between children and teenagers who receive most of the attention and therefore the most support. Those who were youngest in their families talked about being teased and not taken seriously. As for the eldest, they took care of brothers and sisters and complained about being taken for granted, and about not having any privacy for themselves. The girls spoke of their experiences in the classroom where they were separated from their friends, and were expected to assume the responsibility for quieting boys down. They spoke of being chastised for the same behavior that boys got away with, and not being treated fairly in class. They were concerned because they didn't get enough space in the schoolyard and were intimidated by the boys when they tried to participate in sports. They talked about the pressure to be like everyone else and how difficult it was when they excelled at something and were teased by other girls.

Seventh Grade Girls

Seventh grade girls thought about their grungies throughout the week and came to the group prepared with something specific that they wanted to share. They liked to role-play different situations – especially when they could practice different endings, such as saying "no." They also wanted to just sit around and talk. These girls decorated their journals and pasted pictures in them. Often they would read out the parts that they wanted everyone to hear. Throughout the program, they acknowledged how much better they felt about themselves the day after they had come to the group.

Because the girls in seventh grade were at various stages of puberty, they were more self-conscious about their bodies. Some of them were already developed, while others lagged behind their friends. All of them worried about how they looked. During the course of one group I received permission from the girls and their parents to take pictures for a slide presentation. The moment that I brought out my camera, the girls rose *en masse* and went to put on lipstick and comb their hair!

The girls talked a lot about their experiences in school. They felt unfairly punished for behavior that is condoned in boys. They talked about harassment by male teachers who commented on their changing bodies, and by boys who tried to grab their breasts. Some of the girls spoke of themselves as stupid. They were having difficulty in math and were already set to give up.

They spoke about conflicts with parents and step-parents. They expressed the loss that they felt when there was a divorce, and described their conflicting loyalties when they were caught in the middle or forced to choose.

Their greatest concerns were around their developing bodies, their emerging sexuality and their relationships with boys. In seventh grade, girls were already aware of the double standard and of *sluts* and *studs*. They worried about how to hold hands without sweating, and about whether they knew the right way to kiss. They described the "make-out" group that girls with big breasts were invited to join. The girls in the groups were very protective of one another – especially when they saw each other treated badly by the boys.

EIGHTH GRADE GIRLS

Girls in eighth grade saw the group as an appropriate place for them to talk about their personal problems. They referred to it as "therapy," because they felt that talking about things made them feel better. They came equipped with tissues just in case one of them started to cry. Like the girls in sixth and seventh grades, they liked to role-play. Their scenarios were usually built around the intricacies of their interpersonal relationships. While they were inclined to split up into small groups (which they felt were more *personal*), they also liked to just sit around and talk as a whole.

The girls in eighth grade were the most affected by the developmental transitions in their lives – regardless of whether they were in junior high or in the first or second year of high school. The girls spoke about what it was like for them to leave the intimacy of elementary school for the impersonal vastness of the secondary school. They spoke about the changes they saw in their friends, the loss of old friends and their difficulties in making new ones. Some of the girls talked about being intimidated by ninth grade girls who picked on them as they walked to and from school.

They spoke about conflicts in their families as they wanted more freedom and their parents were afraid to let go. They talked about their mothers who expected them to be thin, and their fathers who wanted them to perform. Most of all, the girls talked about the interpersonal dynamics between them, and their fears about over-expressing themselves and taking the risk of losing friends. They spoke about popular girls and cliques and of wanting to fit in. They talked about boys and about dating and about sluts and studs and prudes and of pleasing boys at the expense of themselves.

Dealing with Your Own Grungies

The *Just for Girls* program has now been successfully adapted to many age groups and is used as a resource for other programs that involve girls. The skills that it teaches are not dependent upon participating in a group. Whenever I visit a school class, I try to give girls the tools to help decode their own grungies and find the stories that lie underneath. I've done this as well with adults in my private practice, and with the professionals I've trained. Most girls and women find that it is a relief to be able to silence their negative voice, to put a name to their feelings, and to talk about the things that are real.

You can help girls recognize their grungies and decode the language of fat. All you need is the patience to probe beneath the surface – no matter how frustrating it sometimes seems. You need to become something of a detective in order to decipher their code. Most of all, you need to trust yourself and your instincts, and recognize that there is no right way or wrong way to do this work. If you don't crack the code the first time, you can come back at it again for further attempts. It's a good idea to try out the skills by applying them to yourself first.

Strategies to Consider

- Pay attention to what you are telling yourself. Although the most common grungies are fat, ugly and stupid, we all use them in different ways. Some people say "I feel fat." Others say things such as "If I were smarter or thinner ..." or "I'm so unattractive." There are also other things we tell ourselves when we dump on ourselves. Some people give themselves a grungie when they constantly feel guilty and blame themselves for things that are beyond their control. The first step is recognizing which ones are yours.

- Begin by saying to yourself: "This is not about fat, or ugly or stupid. I know that I'm feeling something else, even if I don't know what it is." We have to take the focus off fat (and ugly and stupid) before we can discover what we are really feeling. Even if you don't know what lies underneath your grungies, the very fact that you are aware of them makes them lose their power. You no longer respond automatically to situations by hitting at yourself.

- Look at the context. Ask yourself what you were doing when you were hit by the grungie. What time of the day was it? Was there anything that you didn't want to do? Were you feeling angry, disappointed, insecure or lonely? These are feelings that most women have difficulty dealing with.

- Describe the circumstances or context when you felt fat, ugly or stupid – but this time leave out the grungie. Try to replace it with a real feeling, something that other people can relate to. For example, the first time you might say "I woke up in the morning and felt fat." Now ask yourself what you would feel if you didn't feel fat. (Stupid, awful, confused, depressed are not allowed!) Try to insert a real feeling or description such as "I woke up in the morning and felt like I didn't want to go to work." At first you may not know what's underneath your grungie. Don't give up. Remember that it takes time to make the connection between feeling fat or ugly or stupid, and something else that is lurking underneath.

- Sometimes women say that they feel fat but there isn't anything underneath it. They say that it's because their clothes don't fit or that they ate too much. Remember that feeling fat always has a negative connotation and is always used as a way of putting ourselves down. Every time we say that we feel fat, what we are really saying is "I don't like my body," which means "I don't like myself," and that is learned behavior. It's also a way of speaking in code. Ask yourself what happened to make you feel fat when you didn't feel "fat" twenty minutes ago.

- If you feel fat all the time (and many women do), just focus on one or two specific incidents. Don't give up. Remember that the reason we speak in code is because some things are just too difficult or scary to say out loud.

- When you do have a sense of what's underneath your grungie, you don't have to do anything directly about it. You don't have to quit your job, leave your husband, or yell at your best friend. It is important for us to know this. Because our society is so focused on "instant" solutions, we think that we have to act immediately every time we have a feeling. We cannot expect ourselves to take action when we are not ready, or don't have the proper skills, or are really scared. But we must guard against silencing what we know, rather than not make any changes.

- Don't repress, express! Many of us think that the only way we can express our feelings is directly to the source. Lots of times it's just too scary and perhaps even inappropriate to yell at our boss or our students or our children's teacher. Find a creative way of telling your story and of getting your feelings out. When we don't express our feelings, they go looping around and around inside our head and we end up giving ourselves grungies. There are many ways for us to express our feelings indirectly:

  - We can find a private place and just talk out loud about what is bothering us.

    – We can say things such as "I'm so angry with John because he forgot my birthday or didn't come home on time. I just want to ..."

    – We can speak to the person symbolically without his or her being there, by saying, "I'm so angry with you John because ..."

    – We can write it out or draw a picture.

- If you start to feel guilty or disloyal or are afraid of hurting the other person, remember that when you express your feelings symbolically, they can't hear you and you don't have to worry about their response.

Once you feel that you have enough practice recognizing your own grungies and decoding the language of fat, you are on the road to being able to help girls when they feel fat.

5

The Influence
of the Media

It's almost impossible for girls to escape the pervasive influence of the media. Children watch an average of four hours of television every day. By the time they reach high school, they have watched approximately 15,000 hours of TV compared to the 11,000 hours they have spent in school.[1] For many, television has become like a surrogate parent. It socializes them, entertains them, comforts them, disciplines them, and tells them what they can and cannot do.[2] When children watch television programs and rock videos, read magazines and listen to music, the relationship they have with the medium is a passive one. They constantly take in copious amounts of images and messages, but because they lack the cognitive skills and life experience to question for themselves what they see and hear and read, it is difficult for them to evaluate the credibility of the information.

Because we rarely watch television or listen to music or read magazines with girls to help them develop critical skills, they believe that what they see and hear and read is true. They internalize the values and attitudes and emulate the behaviors that the media presents

– though these may not be the ones we want them to learn. Television programs such as *Beavis and Butthead* encourage kids to be rude and insulting. *The Mighty Morphin Power Rangers* model physical violence as a way of dealing with conflict and righting what is wrong. Rap music and rock videos on MTV teach boys to call girls "whore," "bitch" and "cunt" – and lead girls to believe that such abusive language is all right and to be expected. Many of the teen magazines encourage girls to focus on their looks and on winning and keeping a boyfriend instead of on living their lives.

As girls make the transition into adolescence, the media ushers them psychologically into a culture based upon and reinforcing unattainable perfection. Shampoo commercials transform women's hair into shimmering cascades rarely seen in real life. Cosmetic companies infer that it is a crime to get old. Sanitary napkins and tampons are used only by young active women – which means that those who are sedentary or disabled never get their periods and that menopause must surely start at twenty-five! Of the 350,000 television and magazine advertisements that these girls have been exposed to in their lives, over 50 percent have stressed the importance of being beautiful and thin.[3]

While the media offers girls images to aspire to, those same images are often not even real. In her video "Slim Hopes: Advertising and the Obsession with Thinness," filmmaker Jean Kilbourne shows how beauty today is a product of technology. Computer imagery alters the size and shape of women's legs, breasts and facial features. Props create illusions. Air brushing takes away any lines or blemishes.[4]

The media is quite rigid in its stereotypes. A recent study of prime time television was carried out by Temple University in Philadelphia for the Screen Actors Guild. It found that men in prime time television outnumber women two to one, that by the time women reach the age of thirty they begin to disappear from major roles on television, and that nine out of ten women on television are under the age of forty-six. When both men and women reach sixty, they begin to disappear altogether.[5] Women who are fat, old, disabled, wear glasses or represent ethnic minorities are rarely major players. They are only occasionally represented, and then just in character parts.

In a workshop I facilitated for the Big Sisters organization, I asked the Big and Little Sisters present to describe their image of the perfect girl or woman. The audience ranged in age from eleven to forty years old. Although the group was racially and culturally mixed, almost all the participants saw the perfect girl or woman as thin, blonde and white. While there are occasionally alternatives to the prevailing image of beauty that girls are offered, they are few and far between. And when girls don't see themselves reflected in the popular culture, they come to believe that something is wrong with them. They never think that something may be wrong with the culture instead. They don't challenge the culture, they try to change themselves. When we don't provide girls with a range of images that celebrate who they are, we allow the media to continue to define how girls come to see themselves. This not only affects girls personally, it also fuels the sexism and racism that society internalizes and in turn passes on to the girls.

When Thin Is In

On a daytime television show, an editor from a popular women's magazine explained how large breasts, perfect bodies and "thin as a finger" dominated the 90s look. As the host recoiled in horror from images of emaciated models flashed on the screen, the editor explained that Chanel's "face" for 1996 was a walking skeleton and that the famous model Wilhelmina ate only twice a week until she died in 1964. While today's models are more muscular and less emaciated, there is no doubt that thin is still in. Because models usually weigh about 20-25 percent less than the average woman in our society, girls who try to look like them are at risk of achieving an unhealthy weight.

The multi-billion-dollar fashion industry panders to an image of clothing by Calvin Klein (and his designer colleagues) for women who are helpless, powerless, subservient, sexually available and dominated by men. They perpetuate the attitude that male authority over women is acceptable. In the world of high fashion, where older means more developed, the demand is for girls who are younger and thinner – such as Corinna, the Bosnian supermodel who was thirteen years old when she was at her peak and who played with dolls between takes. The ideal of beauty that the fashion industry promotes has become so unrealistic that we have children dressing up to look like women and women dressing up to look like little girls.

It's not only in fashion that children have to beat back puberty in order to succeed, but also in such pursuits as competitive individual sports. In both gymnastics and figure skating, two sports that attract a large audience of female viewers, the physical skills have become so demanding that only competitors with prepubescent bodies can succeed. According to Joan Ryan, author of *Little Girls in Pretty Boxes*, the age, height and weight of female gymnasts has steadily decreased in the past forty years.

For the 1992 Olympics in Barcelona, the average U.S. Olympic gymnast was sixteen years old, stood 4 feet 9 inches, and weighed 93 pounds. That year, Russian gymnast Svetlana Boginskaya was nineteen years old, 5 feet 4 inches, and weighed 95 pounds. Although four years earlier she had won two gold, a silver and a bronze medal, she was now too tall and too womanly to explode as high or flip as fast as her 4-foot-6-inch, 70-pound competitors.[6]

In figure skating, 4-foot-8-inch Olympic Gold Medalist Tara Lipinski was only fourteen years old when she competed against the then seventeen-year-old Russian champion Svetlana Slutskaya, who faced the risk of becoming a has-been as she struggled with the changes in balance caused by her developing body. In women's skating, as in gymnastics, women are over-the-hill when they can no longer perform with the flexibility and agility of young girls.

By itself, the media doesn't cause eating disorders. It does, however, intensify whatever preoccupation with food and weight already exists. Girls reinvent themselves in adolescence in order to fit into the male culture. They suppress many vital parts of themselves. Many deal with their distress by turning it against themselves and encoding their feelings and experiences in the language of fat. At the same time that girls begin to feel fat, the culture offers them an ideal shape that is either statistically unattainable or which they can only achieve at the cost of their health. It convinces girls who are going through puberty that not only are the changes in their bodies not normal, but that their bodies are unacceptable or deformed.[7]

At this time when girls are most vulnerable, they are bombarded with the message that everyone should be thin, and that this ideal body shape is attainable – if only they try hard enough. They compare themselves with the images they see, and when they don't measure up they attempt to alter their bodies instead of dealing with the changes in their lives.

Psychologist Karin Jasper describes the ways in which the culture robs us of our sense of self and leaves us powerless to change society's definition of who and how we should be. She looks at how this intensifies our preoccupation with food and weight. According to Jasper, the ads we see for diet programs and for diet foods suggest to women and girls that being in a state of starvation is normal. It is just something to be dealt with by eating copious amounts of diet foods that don't count.

The ads imply that something is wrong with the women who eat real food. They suggest that women should ignore their appetites and trust diet information instead.[8] Many women and girls who are bulimic or who are rigidly dieting follow this advice as if it were a religious practice. Popcorn and rice cakes are sometimes the only foods they eat. Women's magazines tell women that they should cook for others, but they themselves should not eat. Many of the recipes show plates with very little food on them as being normal. While men are encouraged to eat more, a woman who is trying to lose weight is told by such a recipe presentation that she has eaten quite enough. If she is still hungry, it is not because there was something wrong with the recipe but rather that something is wrong with her.

To lessen the influence that the media has on girls, we need to be familiar with what they see and hear. We can begin by watching television and movies with them, by listening to their music and reading their magazines. We need to be familiar with their culture in order to help them recognize, decipher and counter the messages they receive. We can search for books and movies that empower girls and women rather than diminish them. We can provide girls with a wide range of images so they can see that it is all right for them to be who they are. We can help girls build a "bank account" of self-esteem points by continuously giving them specific feedback about their skills, qualities and characteristics. When girls look into the mirror and do not see Tyra Banks, Naomi Campbell or Cindy Crawford, they can fall back on valuing themselves in terms of who they are rather than on how they look.

Strategies to Consider

- Watch television and movies with her. Make a list of the women and girls that you see. How old are they? What are they doing? How do they act? What do they look like? Talk about the messages that these shows and movies are trying to convey.

- Listen to music and watch music videos with her. Discuss what the words mean. Does anybody currently say these things to her? How does that make her feel? What can she do to stop them?

- Make friends with your doctor, dentist and hairdresser. Have them save their old magazines for you.

- Make collages of the different ways in which women and girls are portrayed. Make a collage of the "ideal" women and girls that we see. Make a collage of "realistic" women and girls. Who is included? Who is excluded? Where do you fit in?

- Look at pictures of models. Gather information about the technical processes involved in making someone look this way.

- Look at magazines at your local store or at the grocery store checkout. Count the number of magazines that have diets on their covers. Count the number of magazines that tell you how to please someone else.

- Make a list of girls and women who are your heroes. Add to it as you get more names. Try to be as broad as you can in your selection and not focus just on movie and rock stars. Who are the women and girls that you most admire? What qualities about them do you admire? What are some of the things these women do in their daily lives?

- Make a self-esteem flowerpot. Fill a flowerpot with sand or with kitty litter. Take eight or ten Post-It notes or draw eight or ten daisies. On each one write something that you value about yourself – qualities, characteristics, skills, roles. Tape the "flowers" to straws and stick the straws into the flowerpot.

Notes

1 Barbara Moe. *Coping with Eating Disorders*. New York: Rosen Publishing Group, 1991.

2 Susan J. Douglas. *Where the Girls Are: Growing Up Female with the Mass Media*. New York: Random House, 1994, p. 6.

3 Moe.

4 This was in the video "Slim Hopes: Advertising and the Obsession with Thinness" by Jean Kilbourne (see Resources at the end of this book).

5 [Vancouver] *Sun*, July 2, 1999.

6 Joan Ryan. *Little Girls in Pretty Boxes: The Making and Breaking of Elite Gymnasts and Figure Skaters*. New York: Doubleday, 1995, pp. 64-66.

7 Karin Jasper. "Messages from the Media." Toronto: National Eating Disorder Information Centre Bulletin, March 1994, Vol. 9, No. 1.

8 Jasper.

6

Maintaining Our Connections with Girls

While each stage of female development has its challenges, nothing tests our limits like puberty and adolescence. It's hard not to look at girls and get just a little bit nervous when we see their bodies begin to change – no matter how good a relationship we may have with them now. We look at the world that they are about to enter. We are aware of the adaptations they will be required to make if they want to fit in. We look down the rocky road they are embarking on and view many of the risks that they face with some sobering experiences from our own pasts. We worry about their safety. We are afraid that they will lose their connection with themselves, and that their spirit will get squelched. Most of all we are afraid that the connection we have with our girls will be broken, and that it will never be fixed.

Adolescence today is uncharted territory. When we look back toward our own experiences for guidance, we become aware of how inadequate our personal road maps have become. We are painfully aware of how little they help us in anticipating what lies ahead for girls today. While many of us dieted and worried about our weight when we were younger, eating disorders as such hardly existed or were just on the rise. They certainly were not rampant as they are now. Many of us smoked – and some of us may still do – but more girls are smoking now and they are starting at younger ages. While we experimented with sex in stages as we got older, girls today are having sex earlier than ever before. They may worry about becoming pregnant, as we did. But unlike us, they now run the risk of getting any variety of sexually transmitted diseases that may be chronic or even fatal. And even though we, too, were teased by boys, it was nothing like the sexual harassment that today's girls are experiencing and the level of violence to which they are exposed.

> "I remember how I was with my mother," says Margaret. "The minute I hit puberty, I started to do things behind her back. Right now I have a really close relationship with Jody – but I'm afraid that I'm going to lose it. I'm afraid that when she becomes a teenager she'll start to do the same thing."

> "I don't want Alyson to go through what I went through during adolescence," says Susan. "I was very nervous and very insecure. I didn't think that I could do things. I became really depressed. I don't want her to end up in a situation like that."

> "My biggest fear is for Sarah's safety," says Trisha. "When I was younger I used to take care of my sisters. I'd take them to the beach on the bus all by myself. I won't let Sarah take a bus anywhere by herself."

As girls go through puberty the ties that we have with them as mothers are in danger of becoming severely strained. The girl who was once our constant companion doesn't want to spend time with us anymore. The same girl who once shared her every secret with us begins to tune us out. She turns to her peer group instead for confirmation and validation. She wants to be away, with her friends.

Where once we were the absolute greatest thing in her life, nothing about us is good enough anymore. Every time we try to talk to her, she rolls her eyes at what we say. She judges us through the lens of her own anxiety and through her need to fit in and be like everyone else. While she still has moments when she's proud of us, she also has moments when she feels ashamed. We're different from the women that she admires on TV and in the movies and the music videos. We're either too thin or too fat or too old or too something. We're boring when we don't have whizzy careers, and when we do have them we're blamed because we're never there for her.

Because we are closest to her, we are most often the ones who bear the brunt of her roller coaster ride of hormones. As her sexuality begins to awaken and she becomes interested in boys, she moves even further away from us as she begins to close off certain parts of herself. Though she continues to talk to us about her friends, her schoolwork, and other selected activities in her life, she keeps the things that are most important to her to share only with her friends.

It's often painful when girls begin to seek a replacement for us as the central figure in their lives. It's hard not to feel abandoned, rejected and alone. We feel hurt when girls talk back to us. We assume it is because they no longer care. We don't know how to deal with their anger or the best way to express our own. Because we mistakenly believe this is the way things are supposed to be in adolescence, we deny our feelings or tell ourselves there is something wrong with feeling the way we feel.

At the same time that girls move away from us, we begin to change in how we relate to them. Adolescence was a difficult time for many of us. I don't know anyone who would want to relive their teenage years again. Because they were so painful, we often don't share our experiences and feelings with girls. We think that to do so will burden them. We're afraid that instead of making things better, we will make things worse. We have a mistaken belief that by not sharing our pain with girls, we will somehow be able to spare them theirs.

As girls turn to us to help them make sense of the changes that they are experiencing, we present them with a relational void. Instead of providing them with a much-needed context for what is happening to them, we send them into uncharted territory all alone. They think that they are the only ones who feel the way they do. They think that the feelings they have are wrong. They are sure this is the way they will feel for the rest of their lives. Unless we tell them so, girls don't have any way of knowing that we, too, felt the same way they do – and lived to tell about it.

In our urgency to protect girls from the risks that we know make them vulnerable, we stop talking *to* them and begin to talk *at* them. Instead of sharing ourselves and supporting them through their own process, we try to tell them what to do. As a result, we distance ourselves from them. We get lost in our role as mother, aunt or teacher. We inadvertently recreate with them the kind of power-based relationship that we experience with men. Even though we don't mean to do so, we end up threatening the very connections that we have tried so hard to build up.

Barriers: Recognizing Things That Get in Our Way

We don't interact with girls in a vacuum. Whether we are mothers or other mentors (fathers or other women and men who work with girls), we bring to each and every one of our relationships our own experiences of the world. These are based upon (and colored by) previous relationships with our parents and siblings and other significant people in our lives, on our value systems, on the expectations of society and of other people, and on our unfulfilled expectations and dreams. No matter how much we care about girls and want to do our best, sometimes these other elements can get in our way. As we try to deal with girls' adolescence, it is difficult not to reawaken long-buried feelings and unresolved conflicts of our own. We remember the struggles with our parents, the feeling of not being understood. We remember the restrictions that were placed on our behavior, and how lonely, awkward and different we felt as we tried to adjust and fit in.

> "I was a tomboy," says Trisha. "When I started to go through puberty everything changed. My cousin could do anything he wanted because he was a boy. I was a girl and I was supposed to be nice. I'd get really mad at my parents. They'd let you go so far and then pull you back. I couldn't understand why they did that to me."

> "I was the eldest girl in my family," says Sue. "I went to a private school where there were only seven girls in the class. Until puberty, everyone treated us the same way they treated the boys. Then all of a sudden, the rules changed. My mother made me wear dresses. She told me not to be so smart. My father used to tell me that my mother knew best and left everything up to her. Nobody was on my side anymore."

> "I was really quiet," says Cheryl. "My older sister fought with my mom all the time. I just tried to stay out of her way. I knew that if I did well in school I would please her, and she wouldn't pick on me. So I worked really hard. I didn't have many friends. I felt really alone."

Carrying Our Emotional Baggage

Each time we interact with girls we bring with us our unresolved feelings and conflicts from the past. How much of an impact they have depends upon how well and to what degree we have resolved them. In order for us to open the door to better communication with girls, we need to become aware of our own emotional baggage and the ways in which it influences our lives.

Pushing our buttons: Some situations push our buttons. They trigger an extreme response. We react more strongly and our feelings are much more intense than the situation calls for. Somebody says something and we feel criticized as we were criticized in the past, even if that wasn't their intent. Something someone does can make us so mad that we stay angry for days. We may become so hurt that we are inconsolable.

> "I like to think about myself as a kind of calm person," says Jessica. "But when Bonnie talks back to me I just go nuts. It triggers my memories of all the fights that I had with my own mother. I find myself yelling at her even though I don't want to, and that only makes the situation worse."

Anger that won't go away: Sometimes we seem to be angry with our girls all the time, no matter what they may or may not do. When this happens, it is usually because something else is triggering our feelings. It could be memories from the past, or even something that is happening right now in the present. When we haven't resolved the situation that is at the root of our anger, the anger just won't go away. We deflect it onto the girls and come to believe they are the cause.

> "There is one student in my class, her name is Kelley," says Rachel, "and it seems like no matter what she does, I get angry. It seems like she can't ever do anything right. I know that it's not fair but I can't help it … She reminds me of my sister when she was twelve. My sister was a year older than me and always used to put me down."

When it's hard to hear what they are saying: Sometimes when girls want to talk to us about their concerns we become really uncomfortable and find ourselves tuning them out. It seems hard for us to hear what they are saying. When this happens it means that they have touched upon memories and experiences that were painful to us.

> "I have a hard time when Carmen asks me for advice about her friends," says Marta. "I find that I have trouble listening to her. I was really lonely when I was her age. I didn't have many friends. It's hard for me to relate to what she is saying."

Reacting on her behalf: Sometimes we become overly concerned with the situations that affect girls. We can't get them out of our mind. We lie in bed at night thinking about a fight she had with a friend, a situation where she felt misunderstood, a time where she felt disappointed. It's almost as if we feel the feelings on her behalf. She's already resolved them, but we can't let them go. When her experiences affect us more than they affect her, it's probably because we are reliving events from our own past.

> "Sarah has a friend who is always standing her up," says Trisha. "She'll phone her up and ask her to go to a movie and then when the time comes, she goes with somebody else. Sarah says to me 'Oh that's just Roberta. She does it to everyone.' It makes me so mad. I think about it for days."

Responding to Our Tapes

Imagine that as you are reading this page, you suddenly hear a voice coming from outside telling you that there is a fire. You would probably run out of the room. Now imagine that a tape recorder is sitting on the table in front of you. When it is activated, the same voice tells you that there is a fire. You probably won't react – because you know that what you are hearing is just a tape.[1]

As adults we all carry around internal tapes that we respond to unconsciously. These tapes are made up of our *shoulds* – the messages that we got from our own parents, from our former teachers and from the society in which we live. We *should* do this. We *should* do that. How we respond depends on whether or not we recognize that what we are hearing are prerecorded tapes.

Our *shoulds* keep going off in our head like the tapes in the tape recorder. When we are not aware that what we are hearing are tapes, we respond to them automatically. We do things that we may not even want to do just because we *should* do them. We impose the same *shoulds* upon girls without thinking about where these came from. Often we end up in a power struggle because what we think they should be doing doesn't make sense in the context of their lives and is not what they want to do. Once we start to recognize the nature of our internal taped messages, we have a choice in how we respond. When we are able to interact with girls instead of playing them our tapes, we have a better chance of hearing what they have to say.

The Myth of the Perfect Mother

There was a time when we brought up our children or took care of our nieces and nephews or cousins' children within large extended families. We lived in small communities where everyone kept an eye out for everyone else's child. Because everyone pitched in, the responsibility didn't rest entirely with one person. Changes have taken place in our society, and most of us have left our extended families. We've moved out of our familiar neighborhoods and away from our communities of origin. We began to live in so-called nuclear families made up of a mother and father and kids. Today many of us live in families that are made up of just a mother and her kids.

In the 1950s many families moved to the suburbs, and mothering began to take place in isolation. "Child care" was then categorized as a profession. While mothers were still held responsible for taking care of the kids, a group of male psychologists and doctors told us how we were supposed to do it, which implied that whatever we were already doing was wrong.

Men such as Freud, Piaget, Gesell and Spitz informed us that as mothers we were solely responsible for the success of our children. It was up to us to take care of all their emotional, intellectual, social and physical needs. When Dr. Spock came onto the scene, he found a receptive audience in our growing insecurity. He helped us doubt our instincts and abilities. He told us that the relational way in which we mothered was wrong.[2]

Dr. Spock and his colleagues began a "blame the mother" philosophy of child care that people ascribe to even today. It places unrealistic expectations upon us. It makes us undermine our accomplishment and ourselves and look to others for direction, instead of trusting ourselves. It encourages us to buy into the myth of the perfect mother and to try to live up to ideals that don't make sense and are impossible to achieve.

We all know the perfect mother. She is all-nurturing, all-loving and selfless. She always manages to be there for her kids and is still able to get everything else done around the house. She produces perfect children and always looks good. You can be sure that she isn't anything like us.

Myths of the perfect mother are so pervasive in our culture that women tell me their guilt and sense of inadequacy begins the moment that pregnancy is confirmed. We also internalize these myths in our professional roles. They make us feel that no matter what we do, we won't do it right.

I remember my first year of teaching. I wanted so much to be like the fifth grade teacher in the next class. Her students were always quiet. Her rows of desks were always neatly arranged. Whenever she went to look for something, she always knew where it was. It took me time to recognize that I would never be like her. I was more informal and had lots more energy. I just needed time to find my own style.

When we allow ourselves to be held hostage by these myths of perfection, we never really learn to trust ourselves. We look to other people – to experts – to tell us what to do. We follow their instructions with our heads even if, in our hearts, we know they are wrong.

If we are going to take back some of our power and free ourselves from the expectations of everyone else, we need to stop trying to live up to someone else's notion of perfection. We can begin by recognizing the difference between what is real and what is myth. I am providing you here with just a few examples.[3] You might well discover others as you become more curious about your own belief system.

> *Myth: If I am perfect, everything will be all right.*
>
> *Reality:* No matter how hard we try, none of us can be perfect. We are all a product of our previous experiences and of the society in which we live.

Myth: I am responsible for everything that happens to my daughter. I have the power to make her happy.

Reality: We hold ourselves personally responsible for everything that happens to our girls. We think that if they develop eating disorders, for example, it's because of something that we did or didn't do. The reality is that girls don't grow up in isolation. Social, cultural and economic forces often have a greater impact upon them than we do.

Myth: I can protect my daughter against life's harshness – from its frustrations, losses and despair.

Reality: The hardest part of loving someone is not being able to prevent them from getting hurt. Yet hurt, frustration, loss and despair are all part of being alive. We can't protect girls from life, but we can be there to help them deal with the difficult feelings that are part of being human.

Myth: I should always be gentle, loving, and accept everything she does.

Reality: Girls look to us as examples. They need to know that we can be strong and assertive. That gives them permission to try out a whole range of behavior for themselves. We make girls feel safe when we are able to be honest and set boundaries and limits – even though they may not like it.

Strengthening Our Relationships with Girls

One of the major developmental tasks that girls must accomplish when they reach adolescence is to become autonomous; that is, they learn the skills they need in order to be able to take care of themselves, and to make decisions for themselves. Our society tends to define autonomy through the male perspective of independence and confuses it with separation.

We err in believing the myth that in order for girls to experience themselves as separate from us they must somehow break the connection between us. We have been led to believe that helping girls approaching adolescence separate from us is the thing we should do – even though it goes against everything we believe is right. Girls, too, are taught the myth of separation. They try not to be "dependent" upon us – even when this might be the time they need us most.

Girls are interdependent, as we learned from the section on female development. They develop their sense of autonomy within the context of their relationships. When they move outside this context, they don't feel stronger – they feel more anxious. In our hearts, we know that separation is wrong. The mixed messages in our culture lead us to heighten the tensions between us. Rather than empowering girls and enhancing their psychological growth, we leave them feeling abandoned and alone.

It helps to visualize our relationship with adolescent girls as if they were toddlers first beginning to walk. Imagine they are attached to us by an invisible cord – an elastic band – the length of which is described by their level of comfort and by ours. Each time they wander off away from us and get to a point that no longer feels safe, they come running back for reassurance. Once they re-establish the connection, they wander off again. At the same time that they are pushing us away and heading down the road with their friends, they still want and need to know that we will be there for them when they come back.

It's hard to feel connected with girls during this period. On the one hand we want to hang in there and protect them. On the other we want to pull away because we feel rejected or we need a breather. We struggle with their desire for independence. We don't know how much we should give them. We don't know how to deal with their anger. It's hard for us to trust them or to trust our reactions to them. If we are detached from them or don't set any limits, we stretch the lead too far and we run the risk that it will break. If we impose too many restrictions, we wind it so tightly around us that we end up choking off whatever life exists. It's easier for us to find a balance when we have a clear sense of our own boundaries and can teach girls about theirs.

In *Raising a Daughter*, Jeanne and Don Elium help us understand the concept of *personal boundaries* by describing them in terms of building and respecting fences.[4] Fences let us know where our "yard" begins and ends. Our yard encompasses our sense of ourselves, our hopes and fears, our feelings and our responsibilities to ourselves and to others.

Sometimes we don't share our feelings with girls because we are afraid of hurting them or of being rejected. When we take care of them or take care of ourselves by holding back or by being indirect, we trespass over their fences. We take away their ability to deal with their own feelings and to be responsible for their own reactions. In robbing them of their opportunity to respond we weaken the connection between us. We often try to break down their fences by speaking for them, telling them how they must be feeling or telling them what to do. When girls cross our fences with the same behavior, we recognize how uncomfortable, taken advantage of and angry we feel.

If we are to maintain strong relationships with girls we need to recognize and respect our own fences – our own limits and boundaries – and we need to teach girls to recognize and respect theirs. Teaching girls about their fences and the consequences that come from breaking them allows them to develop internal boundaries (to know what feels right for them), so they can make healthy choices and take responsibility for themselves.

Sharing Ourselves

The greatest gift that we can give girls is to engage with them fully. This means that we learn to listen with our hearts instead of with our heads, that we are honest with them in our responses, and that we begin to share ourselves. Sharing ourselves means that we use our similar experiences as a way of opening up communication, and of letting girls know that we empathize with theirs. Engaging with girls requires us to become aware of our own histories, to learn to negotiate our own emotional land mines, and to try really hard not to get locked into the roles we play.

"I never really knew the effect I had on Clea when I used my 'mother' voice," says Lynn, "until an episode that happened when she was seven. I picked her up after school and we went shopping for decorations for Jakie's party. It was five o'clock. I was tired and money was tight. As we pushed the stroller through the store Clea kept pointing out different things and asking me if we could buy them. Each time I said things like, 'No, we're not getting that,' or 'We can't buy that,' or 'Put that back.' Finally she said to me, 'When you keep saying *no* like that it makes me feel like you're saying all my ideas are bad.' I was taken aback by her response. I said to her, 'I'm not saying that your ideas are bad. It's just that I don't have much money to spend.' 'Well,' she said, 'You should tell me that instead of saying *no*.'"

Sharing ourselves with girls means that we feel free to engage in trouble talk – the kind of interaction that we have with other women in our lives. This doesn't mean that we share experiences that are still emotionally charged, or that we expect them to solve our problems, or that we use them as a sounding board for issues that we are struggling with ourselves. No matter how close we want to be in our relationship to them, we have to remember that we are adults and they are still girls.

Sometimes the things that they talk about make us uncomfortable because our frames of reference and our experiences are very different from theirs. In a grade eight group that I was co-facilitating in an inner city high school, the girls began to talk about what was underneath the language of fat and the times when they felt stupid. Most of the girls had come from war-torn countries. One had seen her parents tortured and killed. As the girls shared their stories, I became aware of how much pain there was in the room, and how uncomfortable and helpless I felt. While a part of me wanted to rush in and try to make the girls feel better, I had to stop myself and take a deep breath. I recognized that the greatest measure of respect that I could show these girls was to listen to their stories and respond as openly and honestly as I could.

Girls respond when they feel connected to us – when we are honest with them about our feelings and our own opinions. By sharing our experiences with them, we validate theirs and form a connection with them that facilitates their growth. We don't always have to know the answer or be patient or agree with their behavior or their points of view. What counts is that we are honest in our interactions with them. The minute that we cease to be ourselves we lose them. When we assume our formal authoritative adult voices we become part of the dominant culture. The girls close down. They begin to act out or, worse, to become "kind and nice."

Female Mentors: The Other Women in Their Lives

When we think of the concept of mentoring, we usually conjure up an image of a well-established adult (usually male) guiding a younger person (also male) along the path of a specific job or career. For women, the concept of mentoring goes much further. It includes showing girls how we handle the personal side of our lives. Mothers are girls' primary mentors. This is a formidable task, requiring mothers to balance their care for themselves with their care for others, setting limits, being clear in their boundaries, and acting on the things that are important to themselves.

Girls also have a whole range of other female mentors. We are teachers, nurses, social workers, child care or youth workers, coaches, Girl Scout or Brownie leaders. We are also older girls, sisters, aunts, cousins and family friends. Because of the relational nature of female development, we can mentor girls even when our connection to them is professional – if we are willing to bring our personal selves into our professional lives. By acting as mentors, we can take some of the pressure off mothers. We can provide girls with support that is less emotionally charged.

"Kate has started to tune me out," says Carly. "I only hope that she chooses wise women to listen to, women who can help her make good decisions."

When girls are very different in personality from their mothers, we can diffuse some of the conflicts by providing them with someone to relate to who might be more like them:

"I'm a get up and go kind of person. I like to get things done right away," says Jean. "Fiona just takes her time."

"Melanie and I are completely different," says Helen. "Part of the problem that I have in dealing with her is that I don't have any kind of recognition of the ways that she is reacting. I don't have any kind of blueprint. Luckily my sister is sort of what she's like, so she is better at figuring out where Melanie is coming from."

We can be mentors to girls when we share an interest with them or have skills in a particular area that their parents don't have. As mentors we can act as role models – not only by showing girls what we do, but also by showing them who we are in a way that relates to them. We can model a way of being that is based on connection and on self-expression, so that girls can retain the positive skills they learned as children and risk losing in the process of growing up.

Whenever I train professional women to work with girls, I encourage them to share their personal selves with the girls. We talk about our own grungies – the times that we felt fat, ugly or stupid during the week. We share our similar feelings. Because many of these women are also mothers, they talk about how they handle issues with their own daughters. The girls in turn like to hear these women's stories because it gives them a mother's perspective on their concerns. It lets them know that other mothers and daughters engage in the same conflicts they do.

Time Out for Yourself

- What was your adolescence like? What was the best experience? What was the worst?

- What were the main issues that you and your parents argued over? Which of these issues come up in your own relationships with girls?

- Lots of times we play a specific role in our families. We can be the pretty one, the smart one, the selfish one, the quiet one, the good one. Who were you? What did that feel like? How does it affect you now?

- Are you labeling the girl in your life? If so, who is she, and what do you do to help keep her that way?

- How did people in your family express their feelings? How did you know that your father was angry? How did you know that your mother was angry? Are you repeating any of these patterns with the girls in your life?

- We all react to certain things. Some situations are harder to handle than others. When you look at your relationships with people (including girls), what buttons get pushed most frequently? How do you respond when they are pushed? What other things get in the way?

- Make a list of your *shoulds*. Try writing them down every day for a week. Whose voice do you hear on the tape? Which of these *shoulds* are you passing on?

- Make a list of your values – the things that are important to you. Which ones are *shoulds* and which are negotiable? Which ones do you think the girl in your life will really need? Where do you meet resistance? How much of this resistance comes from your own unfinished business?

- Make a list of the positive things that you give to girls. Write down the qualities and characteristics that you value about yourself – then act on them.

Time with Each Other

- **Make a commitment to set aside time for just the two of you and honor it.** This will help you remain current with her and show her that she is important to you.

- **Set aside consistent time once or twice a week to deal with complaints.** (Use the strategies outlined in chapter 8 on communication skills.) Declare a truce for the rest of the week. This will break the dynamic that is created in many families: the mother feels that the daughter constantly wants something from her. The daughter feels she is constantly being nagged.

- **Give each other "bouquets."** These can be verbal ones or Post-It notes on the fridge. Praise her accomplishments and qualities. Express your appreciation. Encourage her to do the same with you.

NOTES:

1   Doris Maranda: my former work partner used this tape recorder analogy all the time.
2   Margrit Eichler. *Families in Canada Today*. Toronto: Gage, 1983, p. 137.
3   Evelyn Bassoff. *Mothers and Daughters: Loving and Letting Go*. New York: Plume, 1989, pp. 70-80.
4   Jeanne Elium and Don Elium. *Raising a Daughter: Parents and the Awakening of a Healthy Woman*. California: Celestial Arts, 1994, p. 130.

7

Fathers and Male Mentors

Many men take an active role in parenting. They are involved with their baby throughout the mother's pregnancy. They are present and participate at the birth. They form a strong emotional attachment to their daughters soon after they are born. Those who play an equal role in child care tend to nurture their babies much the same way that mothers do. They speak "motherese," they respond to the baby's cues and they have the same kinds of physiological responses to crying or smiling infants as mothers do.[1]

When the father is not the primary care provider, as relatively few men are, they provide a different kind of nurturing and interaction than mothers when they care for their babies. Fathers are more physical than mothers. They spend less time in taking care of girls by anticipating their needs than in playing with them. As girls grow up their fathers provide them with a male perspective of the world. They teach them a complementary set of skills that are goal-oriented and based upon problem solving and on doing things. When fathers are actively present in their daughter's lives from the beginning, girls tend to develop close and lasting bonds with them.[2]

Supportive fathers generally have daughters with high self-esteem and a sense of well-being. As young women later on, they exhibit more confidence in their relationships with men.[3]

But not all fathers spend this kind of time with their daughters. Many fathers spend their time on the fringe of their families. They leave child-rearing up to their wives. Many men still believe that providing financially for their families is the best way for them to show their love – just like their fathers before them. Because their own self-esteem is tied into what they do rather than who they are, work often comes before the relationships in their lives. Although they may want to have relationships with their daughters, they often lack the skills.

Fathers who are distant with their daughters are more likely to be less understanding and less willing to listen to their concerns.[4] As girls grow up, these fathers are more likely to impose and reinforce society's standards instead of supporting their girl in being the person she really is. When girls learn to not expect much from their fathers, they don't ask for much from any of the men in their future. When they can't ask for what they want directly, they learn to be indirect, manipulative and coy.[5]

Fathers become increasingly important to girls as they grow up. Girls between the ages of eight and twelve want to be included in their father's world. They want to spend time with him and share his interests and activities. They want to be his pal. Many girls feel closest to their fathers during this stage of their development – just before puberty.

This is the time when they are androgynous and are least hampered by societal expectations,[6] so fathers are most comfortable with them now because they can relate to them like boys. There is nothing wrong with this. When fathers and daughters can share common interests and activities, it's easier for them to sustain their relationship throughout the changes that lie ahead.

When girls begin puberty their relationship with their father begins to change. According to psychologist Margo Maine, author of *Father Hunger*, many girls begin to experience *father hunger* – a deep, persistent desire for emotional connection with their fathers.[7]

Many fathers are uncomfortable with their daughters' awakening sexuality. Fathers can find themselves sexually aroused when their daughters' bodies begin to change – especially if they have been otherwise distant in their daughters' lives. Most fathers don't know what to do with these feelings. They don't know how to interact with their daughters now that they perceive them in sexual terms.

Rather than deal with their feelings, many fathers withdraw, to distance themselves from what they see as a potential problem. Many girls feel rejected by the primary man in their lives just when they are beginning to experience themselves as women. During the time when girls are renegotiating their relationships with their mothers, they feel this loss of their fathers' support most deeply, which causes them a whole lot of pain.

> "My dad is never home," says Karen. "He never comes home at night before midnight. If I ask him how his day was he grunts and tells me that he has to take care of his patients. He doesn't ask about me. He just tells me what to do."

> "My dad missed my birthday and graduation," says Marianne, fighting back her tears. "It really hurt. He spends two weeks with us in the summer and buys me a fancy bike and things like that. He thinks that makes up for a whole year."

Girls wonder what they have done to cause this loss of the relationship with their fathers. Because they come to think that there is something wrong with the way they are, they reinvent themselves in order to make themselves more acceptable. Many encode their anger in the language of fat and try to change their bodies by dieting. When fathers are critical of their daughters' weight, or of the amount of food that they eat, this makes it more difficult for girls to accept their changing bodies and reinforces their preoccupation with food and weight.

As girls become women, they look to their fathers for validation of their worth. If their father is disrespectful of their mother, if he constantly criticizes her and puts her down, girls are faced with a dilemma. They are torn between their instinctive loyalty to and identification with their mothers, and their need for connection with their fathers. They often become allies with their fathers against their mothers. To keep their fathers' approval, they begin to disown the female parts of themselves.

Fathers walk a fine line between objectifying girls and validating their femininity. Some fathers try to help their girls fit into the mainstream culture by encouraging them to be attractive and making comments about their weight. While we all need someone who thinks that we are beautiful, it's harmful when that beauty is equated with our body shape. Instead, give girls positive feedback about things that they do not have to change such as, "I like that sweater because it matches the color of your eyes," "That color looks good on you," "I like that dress – it's an interesting design," or "I like when you pull your hair back." Focus on things such as the strength of their bodies and on those things they can do well.

Most fathers want the best for their daughters. In a world where there are a lot more options opening up for women, they try really hard to help their daughters succeed. Because they are products of male development, they offer encouragement that is goal-oriented and which sometimes has a negative effect and is seen as criticism. Telling girls to try harder or telling them that they can be anything they want makes them feel that there are expectations they may not be able to meet – as if who they are is not good enough.

> "My dad constantly criticizes me," says Janie. "He keeps telling me that he always got 90s in school and so did my mom. He thinks I should be doing better. He says that I am not working hard enough."

Girls respond to feedback that takes into account *process* as well as the *goal*. This means that we first need to acknowledge what girls have already accomplished – how they have progressed to where they are. We have to let them know that we can see how hard they have worked. Once we have provided them with that context, then they are ready to listen to suggestions and are more open to what we might say.

It is important for a father to understand about the differences in male/female development – to know where on the gender continuum he and his daughter fall. While there are many things that he can teach her about male culture, he must also take time to learn about hers and communicate in her language. Fathers must value the relational and nurturing parts of their daughters. To do that they must value these qualities in themselves.

Fathers can remain connected to their daughters by spending time interacting with them, doing things with them and remaining a part of their lives. They can help girls withstand some of the societal expectations. They can help them be assertive and take their stand. They can encourage girls in sports and academics. They can model good male-female relationships that are built upon equality and respect.

Some fathers are getting together to learn how to strengthen their relationships with their daughters. Dads and Daughters is a non-profit organization that works to connect fathers so that they can learn from each other and can work to make the world a place where girls are respected for who they are and not for how they look.

> "My dad makes us breakfast," says Laurie. "Even when he comes home late, he comes into my room to say hi and to ask me how my day has been. It helps, even though he is busy and I'd like to see him more."

Time Out for Yourself

If you are a father (or a male mentor) who is reading this book, you have by now probably learned a whole lot about your relationships with women and about the world of girls. You might find it helpful to look into your own attitudes and behavior and to learn a little more about yourself:

- What was your relationship with your own father like? How close or how distanced was he? How would you have wanted things to be different?

- How are you repeating the same pattern in your relationships with girls?

- Look at your own concept of masculinity. How does it contribute to how close or how distanced you are?

- Look at your image of the perfect woman. How do your own attitudes affect your relationship with your daughter and your aspirations for the kind of woman she will be?

- How important is it to you for your daughter to fit society's definition of beauty, or to be thin? How do you convey this to your daughter?

- How do you help her feel good about herself?

- How hard is it for you to truly listen to your daughter without trying to fix her?

 ## Time with Each Other

- **Set aside time just for the two of you.** Try to truly listen to her without telling her what to do. Validate her uniqueness.

- **Be active with her.** Ride a bike, go for a walk, etc. Encourage her to be active.

- **Plan a project together.** The best sharing often comes from doing things together.

- **Get involved in her activities.** This lets her know that you care and gives you a context for what is happening.

Notes

1   M.E. Lamb, A. Frodi, C. Hwang, M. Frodi and J. Steinberg. "The Effects of Gender and Caretaking Role on Parent-Infant Interactions" in R. Emde and R. Harmon, eds. *Development of Attachment and Affiliation Systems*. New York: Plenum, 1982.

2   Irene P. Stiver. "Beyond the Oedipus Complex: Mothers and Daughters" in Judith Jordan et al. *Women's Growth in Connection: Writings from the Stone Center*. New York: Guilford Press, 1991, pp. 105-109.

3   Mary Pipher. *Reviving Ophelia: Saving the Selves of Adolescent Girls*. New York: Ballantine Books, 1994, pp. 118-119.

4   Pipher.

5   Jeanne Elium and Don Elium. *Raising a Daughter: Parents and the Awakening of A Healthy Woman*. California: Celestial Arts, 1994, p. 94.

6   Emily Hancock. *The Girl Within*. New York: Fawcett Columbine, 1989, p. 25.

7   Margo Maine. *Father Hunger: Fathers, Daughters and Food*. California: Gürze Books, 1991, p. 3.

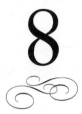

Building Good Communication Skills

Communication refers to any behavior that carries a message to someone else. It doesn't even have to be intended, but once somebody else receives the message, communication has taken place. Just because we send a message doesn't guarantee that it will be received or that the other person will interpret it the way that we intended. Even if there is a response, it may not be the one that we want. Communication needn't be verbal. My cat, Olivia, communicates volumes just by the way she sits by her feeding dish.

Good communication is made up of clear messages and receptive responses. It means that we can talk and listen to each other in such a way that we understand what it is like to stand in the other person's shoes. It doesn't mean that we have to agree with her. It doesn't mean that we have to do what she wants when she wants it. It means that we can each understand how and why the other person feels the way that she does. Good communication opens the door for negotiation. It leaves us feeling connected to each other even though we may disagree.

Sometimes our messages are indirect or incomplete or inaccurate. When we bang the kitchen cupboards, slam the bedroom door, sing in the shower, or let our shoulders droop and our bodies sag as we sit on the couch, we are sending messages to the people around us. We provide people with hints and hope that they will be able to guess what we are trying to say. Sometimes we send messages telepathically. We think that if people love us they will be able to read our minds, and then we are surprised and hurt when they can't.

Sometimes our messages are constructed along the lines of a legal brief. We provide evidence of every little thing the person has ever done wrong before – as if documenting previous transgressions gives us the right to feel the way we do now. So it's not surprising that when we try this form of communication, the other person either hurries to defend herself or withdraws.

Bad communication is a dead end. It doesn't leave us with anywhere to go. Interactions like the ones cited below create roadblocks. They trigger blame, defensiveness and guilt.

> "I waited up all night for you! I couldn't sleep. Don't you know that I have a big appointment today? Why can't you be more considerate?"

> "If you really cared about me, you'd pick up your clothes without my asking. You'd try to make things easier for me."

> "You never tell me where you are going. Last week you went out with Shirley and you came home way past your bedtime. The week before I had to call all your friends to see where you were."

Practicing Responsive Listening

Our communication skills determine how painlessly we get through our girls' adolescence and how much support we are able to give them. There are two kinds of communication. The first is goal-oriented and deals with giving and receiving information. This is primarily what school is all about. In this chapter, I have concentrated on the second kind – which is process-oriented and deals with building and strengthening the connections between us.

Good communication skills begin with listening. The way that we listen to people influences the kind of interaction we have with them and how much they are willing to share. When we try to give advice, solve problems or tell people what to do when they are not ready for it, they will either stop speaking, agree and then tune us out, or storm off feeling misunderstood. When we can show other people empathy or support and can validate or confirm what they are saying, then they feel listened to and tend to open up to us more.

To practice responsive listening:

- Focus on the verbal and nonverbal meanings of the message.

- Let the other person know that you are paying attention to her. You can nod your head, maintain eye contact, and make sounds such as "ah" and "hah."

- Acknowledge and respond to both the content and the emotional undertones of what she is saying.[1]

Let's look at some examples of how responsive listening works:

> *Sarah: "I got a D on my exam in geography. I really studied for it. That Mrs. Jones is not fair."*
>
> *Responsive Listening:* "It sounds like you really studied for your test and only got a D (Content). That must be really disappointing for you. It sounds like you're angry with Mrs. Jones (Feeling)."

> *Lisa: "Sally ignored me in school today. Now she's hanging out with Mary. She doesn't want to be my friend anymore."*
>
> *Responsive Listening:* If Sally was my friend and she was hanging out with someone else (Content), I'd feel really hurt (Feeling). Is that the way you feel?"

When girls feel heard, they feel that their opinions and feelings are of worth, and that we are accepting and not judging them. This increases the level of trust that they have with us and encourages them to continue sharing their feelings with us.

Checking Out Our Perceptions

Two of the greatest stumbling blocks that we face are our mistaken beliefs that we perceive and observe people in an unbiased way, and that if we know them well we can consistently interpret their behavior. The reality is that each time we communicate with someone else we do so through a lens or filter that is colored by our experiences and by our race, culture and gender. Even our own moods color our interpretations. When we are feeling irritable or discouraged we often tend to perceive other people's behavior a lot differently than when we are feeling happy and secure. We also make the mistaken assumption that the other person's behavior has to do with us – if they seem unhappy or tune us out, it must be because of something that we have done.

Good communication involves double-checking and confirming our perceptions. To do this you need to:

• Describe the behavior.

• Give your interpretations of the other person's thoughts and feelings.

• Ask if your perceptions are accurate.

Checking out our perceptions means asking questions such as:

"You slammed the door when you came in (Description). I wondered if you were angry (Interpretation). Are you ?"

"I'm not sure from the way that you are talking (Description), whether you are hurt or angry (Interpretation). Are you feeling either?"

"You seem awfully quiet today (Description). Is it because you are worried about the test that you have in math (Interpretation)?"

Giving Feedback: Using "I" Instead of "You"

Whenever we begin our communication with "you" it's almost as if we're pointing a finger at the other person. We say things like "You didn't do the dishes" or "You said you were going to call and you didn't" or "You always spend too much time on the phone." Finger pointing makes the other person defensive. She can't take it in, so we don't get our message across. Good communication begins when we replace our "you" with "I." It addresses the problem by describing the behavior and takes the emphasis off the worthiness of the other person.

When you want to get the message across in such a way that the other person will listen:

• Describe the behavior. The aim is to give the other person a clear idea of what she did in that specific incident that made you react.

• Describe the feelings that you had. This makes use of the "I" statement. It lets the other person know the emotional impact that the behavior had on you.

• Describe the effect or outcome to let the other person understand how the behavior affected you personally.

Let's look at some examples of how this works:

Issue: "When you stayed out late last night and didn't call me (Description), I was really worried (Feeling). I didn't know where you were (Effect). I thought that something terrible had happened to you.

Issue: "When you leave your clothes all over the floor (Description), I get angry with you (Feeling). The mess really bothers me. When I am under a lot of pressure and things are not in order I get anxious (Effect)."

When the other person responds:

- Listen with curiosity. Try not to plan your answer in advance. Good listening has nothing to do with winning or with planning a rebuttal. It has to do with keeping the communication open and alive.

- Ask yourself if there are parts of her story where you can see how she might have felt the way that she did. You may not have felt the same way, but you respect the way that she feels. In this step, all you want to do is see if you can understand her feelings and her point of view – even though your perception of the incident might be very different.

- Acknowledge her feelings. Let her know that you can see how she might have felt the way she did.

- Tell your side of the story. Use "I" messages to get your point of view across.

Most of us learned our communication skills when we were young. It takes time to change them. It also takes a while to build up the necessary trust so that we can say what we feel without needing to protect ourselves from getting criticized or blamed. Good communication takes a lot of practice. When we want to give people feedback, it's best to start out with something small – such as saying "I" instead of "you" every time we want to say something about ourselves. Then we can graduate to the issues that are not so emotionally charged. Good communication means that we both know the rules and make sure that we both obey them. This ensures that when we fight, we fight fair. Once we've had enough practice, we're better able to deal with the major conflicts when they arise.

Dealing with Defensiveness

Sometimes when we try to get our message across, the other person has difficulty hearing us because her fear of being criticized gets in the way. When people are defensive, we sometimes tend to get caught up in responding to their reaction instead of staying with what we want them to hear. Our conversations are often like this one:

Gina: "When I came home from work today it really bothered me that you left a mess in the kitchen."

Stacey: "It's not my fault. Michelle phoned and I had to talk to her."

Gina: "Well you could have told her to call you back later."

Stacey: "You don't want me to talk to Michelle. You don't want me to have any friends."

Gina: "That's not true. I do want you to have friends."

Stacey: "See, it's always what you want and never what I want."

Gina: "That's not true. I gave you money yesterday when you went out with Michelle."

When you are dealing with someone defensive, it is important to:

• Keep your message simple. Describe the behavior and how you feel.

• Let the other person know that you are not criticizing her.

• Don't respond to her content. Instead, keep repeating your own message until you feel that she hears you. Even if you have to do this five or six times, don't give up.

Let's look at how Gina could have been more effective in her communication with Stacey:

Gina: "When I came home from work today it really bothered me that you left a mess in the kitchen."

Stacey: "It's not my fault. Michelle phoned and I had to talk to her."

Gina: "I'm not trying to criticize you but it really bothers me that you left a mess in the kitchen."

Stacey: "You don't want me to talk to Michelle. You don't want me to have any friends."

Gina: "It really bothers me that you left a mess in the kitchen."

Stacey: "You're always nagging me.

Gina: "No, it really bothers me that you left a mess in the kitchen."

Stacey: "See, it's always what you want and never what I want."

Gina: "No, it really bothers me that you left a mess in the kitchen."

Stacey: "I'm sorry. I'll try to clean up tomorrow."

Dealing with Conflict

It is impossible to have a relationship with someone without ever running into conflict. No matter how much we love the girls in our lives there are bound to be times when we don't see things the same way. When I ask mothers and daughters to talk about their major sources of conflict, their answers are usually the same. Girls want more freedom as they move into adolescence. They want to go off and hang out with their friends. They want to stay out later. The mothers are afraid of what will happen if they allow this.

> "Bonnie and I fight a lot over her independence," says Jessica. "She wants to go off and do things on her own. I know that I should let her but I'm really afraid. I know that this is a time when we have to let go and let them do things on their own. But I have to tell you, I am really scared."

We tend to treat girls and boys differently during adolescence. We see adolescence as a time of self-discovery and increasing independence for boys. When boys begin to challenge authority, we reward it as positive, masculine behavior. It's a sign that they are learning to stand on their own two feet.

As girls approach adolescence, we try to restrict their activities in an effort to protect them from physical danger. When girls try to challenge or question our authority, we tend to put them down.[2] Our society rewards girls for being "good" and "nice," which leaves them no way to be "bad" and challenge the adaptations imposed upon them. Girls trying to assert themselves are often accused of being selfish and inconsiderate. We are afraid of their anger because we have never learned to deal with our own.

Conflict can be scary, but it is also healthy. Studies show that girls who grow up in families that allow conflict have higher self-esteem and a greater capacity for deep, fulfilling relationships with others.[3] Although most of us would like to make conflict go away, engaging with girls in honest conflict helps build the trust between us. It gives girls skills that they can take into the world.

Strategies for Resolving Conflicts

- Look at yourself first. To what extent do your reactions come from having your buttons pushed or from the extra baggage that you are still carrying around from your past?

- Examine your "shoulds." Ask yourself why your point of view is so important. Ask yourself whom you are trying to please.

- Share yourself. Separate your fears into what's real and what's imagined. Sometimes girls will do things behind our back if it is really important to them, or if it is a part of their peer culture. Sharing your fears gives girls permission to talk about theirs, and leaves the door open for further communication.

- Check out your perceptions.

- Practice "I" messages.

- Listen with understanding.

- Stay with the specific issue. It's not fair to use past transgressions as ammunition in the current conflict.

- Avoid generalizations. Statements like "you always" or "you never" leave you both with no place to go.

- Speak for yourself. We sometimes use statements like "everyone says that ..." in order to build our case. Try not to bring in other people. Be specific and speak for yourself.

- Avoid comparisons. Don't compare the other person to someone else, such as: "Mary's mother lets her ..." or "Jennie's daughter always ..."

- Don't make assumptions. We often make assumptions about other people's behavior. Then we respond not to the person, but to the assumption that we made. When I first started my private practice, I developed and facilitated workshops with a partner. One day, after Doris and I dealt with a conflict that came up between us, I heard her sniff. I assumed that she was holding back tears and that she was still angry. As the sniffing continued, I became really uncomfortable – because I didn't want to deal with any more conflict. I tried to ignore her behavior, but finally I asked her if she was still angry. "Oh no," she replied, "it's just that my sinuses are really bothering me today." I learned from this experience that we never really know what goes on with other people until we check things out.

- Clarify the language. We not only make assumptions about people, we also think that we mean the same things. Take the statement "I want to date," for example. When Bonnie told Jessica that she wanted to date, what she meant was that a whole group of kids were going to a movie and she wanted to sit with a particular boy. What Jessica heard was that Bonnie wanted to go out alone with a boy. She was afraid that Bonnie would get "boy crazy." Her schoolwork would suffer. She would become sexually active at twelve. The further Jessica's imagination took her, the more afraid she got and the more rigid she became.

- Make sure that you respect the rules. Discuss how you should handle the conflicts between you. Establish what the rules are to be and make sure that both of you observe and/or enforce them.

- Define the conflict as a mutual problem. A mutual problem is a win-win situation where both people stand to gain.

- Create a supportive climate. Try not to increase her anxiety. It helps if you tell her that you are sure that the conflict can be resolved and reassure her that you are not trying to blame or criticize her.

- Set aside uninterrupted time to talk. This confirms for both of you that your relationship is important, and that you have a commitment to resolve the issues before you. It's hard to listen to each other when other people are interrupting, interfering or taking sides.

- Call time-outs. Not all conflicts can be resolved right away, especially if they are about emotionally charged issues. It sometimes helps to call a time-out when you realize that you are going around in circles and that your feelings are really strong. Calling a time-out, and rescheduling for another day, allows both of you to cool off. This gives you time to reflect and reconsider the other person's point of view.

- Write a letter. Sometimes we are simply afraid to say certain things to the other person. We are afraid that they won't listen or that they will have a really strong reaction. Writing a letter gives them an opportunity to have their reaction and then go back and read it again. Remember that the same rules apply to writing letters as to verbal communication. Be specific and talk about yourself.

Our Feelings

Feelings are the emotional and physical ways in which we learn to respond to our own thoughts and to what goes on in the world around us. They constitute the inner voice, or guide, that provides us with information that helps us understand ourselves better. They tell us what we like and what we want, what is safe and what is not, and about our reactions to other people. When we feel love and affection for someone, for example, we want to move closer to them. When we feel fear, we move away from whatever is causing it. Anger and hurt tell us that we have a problem with another person that has to be fixed. When we feel disappointed, it's because we wanted something and didn't get it. When we feel joy we feel that we are on top of the world.

We have the potential from birth to develop a whole range of feelings, and to experience different degrees of intensity for each one. It's as if every one of us comes equipped with every single feeling imaginable and keeps these feelings in a special "feeling" box. As we grow up, our families and the society in which we live teach us that there are good feelings and bad feelings. We learn that some feelings can be expressed just a little bit, and other feelings can be expressed a lot. Girls are encouraged to let out just the positive feelings, and then only those that have to do with fostering their relationships with others. Girls can feel love, compassion and empathy. Feelings such as anger, jealousy, sexuality, competition and competence are supposed to be stuffed back in the box. Disappointment is a very difficult feeling, because we are taught that if we are disappointed, we shouldn't have wanted what we obviously didn't get. While anger and hurt are different sides of the same coin, most of us learn to express the hurt – but the anger has to be repressed.

The taboo against expressing our anger is so strong that most of us don't even know when we are angry. We find out from some of the things that we tell ourselves, or some of the things that we do. When we can identify our anger, we quickly transform it into something else. Because we are held hostage by the tyranny of kind and nice, we turn our anger against ourselves. Because it is difficult for us to deal directly with the person or situation that triggered the feeling, we say that we are angry with ourselves. Instead of feeling and expressing our true feelings, we encode them in the language of fat. We feel fat and ugly and/or stupid. Sometimes our anger seeps out, and we express it indirectly. We become sarcastic or hostile or we withdraw from the other person. Sometimes our anger boils over, and we attack the other person verbally or physically.

Because we have difficulty with our own anger, we can't handle the anger of others. Yet, like our other feelings, our anger is energy. If we don't deal with it directly, there's no other healthy means of making it go away. Anger is a gift when it is expressed respectfully. It's a way of telling people that you care enough about the relationship between you that you want to set things right.

Holding Back Our Feelings: Taking Care of Someone Else

Girls struggle with the same dilemma that we do: How do you have a relationship with someone and still take care of yourself? They have difficulty balancing their own needs with the fear of hurting or angering someone else. In the process of holding back their feelings, they begin to withdraw. In one grade eight group, Karen and Eva had to deal with the fact that while both of them wanted it, only one of them got the part in the play. Eva arrived at the group first, and Karen came half an hour later.

Eva: "Ooh, I'm so mad that Karen got the part. She's not here right now. She went to pick up her script. I'm not in the play so I came on time. I guess I'm jealous, but I'm trying to be nice so that I don't hurt her feelings. The worst part is going to be when she asks me to help her with her lines. I'm trying to feel happy for her because she's my friend. I *should* help her. I don't know if I can say this to her outside the group, but if she comes today I will."

Karen comes in with her head down and her shoulders hunched. Eva, true to her word, tries to tell her how she feels. Instead of talking about her jealousy, she begins with a litany of all the things about Karen that bug her.

Karen: "I didn't want to come today. My stomach has been upset all day. I didn't want to say anything about the play. I know that you feel bad. I don't want to make it worse. I'm afraid that you won't be my friend."

When the girls are able to identify their feelings and to talk honestly about them, and when they learn basic conflict resolution and communication skills, they are able to repair the rifts between them. This is not the case most of the time, unfortunately. When we are hurt or angry or jealous and can't express our feelings, we tend to withdraw. Most of us carry around a secret list. On it are the ten (or more) worst things about ourselves that we would never want anybody to find out. When people withdraw from us, and don't tell us why, we imagine right away that it's because of the things on our list. Instead of hurting someone with our honesty, we make them victims of their own fears by our withdrawal. In the end that hurts them even more.

 ## Time Out for Yourself

- Which feelings are easy for you to feel?

- Which ones are difficult?

- How do you deal with your feelings?

- How do people know that you are angry or that you are hurt?

- What are the ten worst things that you wouldn't want anyone to find out about you?

- Explore your feelings. Make a list of all the feelings that you can imagine. "Angry at myself," "stressed," and "depressed" are garbage can feelings – because they combine a whole lot of specific feelings that we haven't learned to separate out and identify.

  – Which feelings are you comfortable feeling?

  – Which feelings make you feel like something's wrong?

  – Which feelings do you think you need more practice with?

- Talk about how you express anger. You can help each other figure out the clues. Where can you feel anger in your body? What happens to the energy when we can't let it out? What are some of the ways that people express their anger badly? Why don't these ways work?

- Practice expressing anger. Sometimes when we are angry it is too scary to tell someone directly. Even though you might feel silly at first, try talking to someone who isn't there. You can do this by talking to a pillow or a chair or talking out loud or just writing things down. There is no right thing to do. The most important thing to remember is that it is better to get it out, in whatever way works for you, than to let it fester inside where it ends up being turned against yourself.

- Hold a dead flower ceremony. Girls love rituals. Hold a dead flower ceremony to get rid of your negative feelings. Collect a bunch of dead flowers. Put a wastepaper basket in the middle of the room. Stand next to the basket and imagine the person the dead flower is meant for. Describe their behavior out loud and tell them how that made you feel. Tell them what you would want to say to them if you didn't have to worry about their feelings, or about being regarded as a nice person. Throw the dead flower into the basket and let the feelings go.

Notes

1   William B. Gudykunst, Stella Ting-Toomey, Sandra Sudsweeks and Lea P. Stewart. *Building Bridges: Interpersonal Skills for a Changing World.* Boston: Houghton Mifflin, 1995.

2   Dr. Carol J. Eagle and Carol Colman. *All That She Can Be: Helping Your Daughter Achieve Her Full Potential and Maintain Her Self Esteem during the Critical Years of Adolescence.* New York: Simon and Schuster, 1993, pp. 25-26.

3   Alexandra G. Kaplan, Nancy Gelason and Rona Klein. "Women's Self Development in Late Adolescence" in Judith Jordan, et al. *Women's Growth in Connection: Writing from the Stone Center.* New York: Guilford Press, 1991, p. 127.

PUTTING OUR SKILLS TO WORK

Girls' Issues,
Girls' Lives

9

Puberty

Puberty refers to all of the physical changes that happen inside and outside of a child's body as it transforms into an adult body with the capacity to reproduce. It marks the beginning of adolescence, the stage of development that occurs between childhood and adulthood. At a biologically determined time, the pituitary gland sends a message to the sex glands and puberty begins. In girls, the ovaries sharply increase their production of the female hormone estrogen. In boys, the testes increase production of the androgens, especially testosterone. These hormones are responsible for the sexual maturation that will take place over approximately the next two years.

While girls and boys will undergo many physical changes during puberty, the most dramatic are those that involve sexuality. The internal organs necessary for reproduction (what we call the primary sex characteristics) enlarge and mature, making girls and boys capable of sexual reproduction. In girls, the primary sex characteristics are the ovaries, uterus, fallopian tubes and vagina. Menstruation is the chief sign of sexual maturity. In boys, they are the testes, penis, prostate gland and seminal vesicles. Sexual maturity is determined by the presence of sperm in their urine.

Hormones also stimulate the secondary sex characteristics. These are the physiological signs of sexual maturity that don't directly involve the reproductive organs. Secondary sex characteristics include the breasts of girls and the broad shoulders and facial hair of boys – as well as changes in both sexes in the voice, the texture of the skin, and pubic and body hair. As secondary sex characteristics begin to appear, girls and boys begin to look like mature women and men.

During puberty, girls and boys gain roughly 20 percent of their adult height and 50 percent of their weight. Their skeletal mass, heart, lungs, liver, spleen, pancreas, various glands and sexual organs (including the uterus in girls) double in size. Even their eyes grow faster, causing an increase in nearsightedness during this time. Their bodies begin to change shape as they grow bigger, so that boys get the shoulders and girls get the hips.

Girls and Puberty

Our growth is slow and steady throughout childhood until we reach adolescence. We grow about 2½ inches and 6½ to 7½ pounds each year. Girls and boys are usually the same height at nine years of age, but girls weigh more. When girls are about nine-and-a-half years old, their bodies begin to grow at a much faster rate. This adolescent growth spurt signals the beginning of puberty. Girls usually enter puberty when they are about ten – two years earlier than boys. Every individual is different, so some girls may begin puberty as early as seven and others as late as fourteen. Puberty usually lasts about two years, although some girls can be finished in a year and a half while others may take up to six years.

Girls grow about 10 inches in height during the years when puberty takes place. They grow faster during this period than at any other time in their lives with the exception of infancy. They gain about 3½ inches in the first year, then the growth rate slows down. Around the time girls have their first menstrual period, their growth averages 1 to 2 inches a year. Girls reach their full adult height within one to three years after their first period, when increased levels of estrogen in the bone cells prevent them from dividing as rapidly as before.

During this period of rapid growth girls may sleep longer at night and may nap after school. This is because the hormones that cause them to grow are secreted at a much greater level when they sleep. Girls also develop a tremendous appetite. This ensures that the body has enough fuel to accommodate the changes that are taking place.

When girls are about ten, they begin to develop breasts and body hair. Breast development is very gradual and takes an average of four-and-a-half years and sometimes even longer. The first sign of change in the breasts is when they begin to bud. Buds are the mounds that form (or *bud*) from the milk ducts and fat tissue under the nipple and areola. The nipple can get larger before or after the breast buds begin to form. The areola (the part around the nipple) gets wider, and both the nipple and areola get darker in color. These changes may continue as puberty progresses and girls' breasts get rounder and fuller and begin to stand out more. Changes in the shape and color of the areola and nipple happen regardless of breast size. They are better indicators of sexual maturation than is breast size alone.

Some girls begin to grow pubic hair before their breasts begin to bud. Pubic hair helps keep clean the area between the labia majora (the outer lips of the vagina) and protects the sensitive area between them. The first pubic hairs are silky and just slightly curly. Later, they become dark, thick, coarse and tightly curled. After their breasts have begun to bud, their pubic hair has started to grow, and they have had their first menstrual period, girls begin to develop hair under their arms and sometimes on their upper lip.

Girls develop a distinctly female smell during puberty. Their sweat glands become more active and for the first time in their lives their perspiration begins to smell like adult sweat. As their vaginal lining thickens, it begins to produce secretions that also have a distinct odor. Girls become aware of the mild odor of menstrual blood. At this stage of puberty the texture of the skin begins to change and the oil glands become more active. For many girls, the oily skin leads to pimples and blackheads and sometimes even to acne, but this is more common in boys.

By the time that girls have finished puberty they will have doubled their weight. This means that on the average they will have gained between 40 and 50 pounds. (Remember that this doesn't take place all at once but over a period of several years.) This weight is added to all areas of their bodies, especially their breasts and hips, in the form of fat. Fat gain at this time plays a role in regulating the female hormones estrogen and progesterone, which are necessary for menstruation and pregnancy. For women, the percentage of body fat is one and a half to two times greater than it is for men. Because muscle growth occurs at an earlier age in girls, this is the one time in their lives that they are much stronger than boys.

The Menstrual Cycle

Menstruation is the monthly shedding of the tissue from the lining of the uterus or womb. The first time that a girl gets her period is called menarche. Most girls don't ovulate during these first twelve to eighteen months. However, because individual girls' bodies and cycles are different, girls who do ovulate early are able to conceive soon after they get their first period.

The menstrual cycle is the time from the first day that girls get their periods to the next time that they begin to bleed again. While the average menstrual cycle is twenty-eight days, it can vary between twenty-one and thirty-five days. While each girl will eventually develop her own lifetime pattern, menstrual cycles generally tend to be irregular during adolescence.

The length of a menstrual period is an individual thing. While the average period lasts about five days, it can be as few as two and as many as seven days and vary in duration from month to month and year to year. The amount of blood also varies from one to eight tablespoons and, in some cases, to as much as one cup. Girls and women can have both light and heavy periods throughout their lives. The blood and tissue that make up the menstrual flow may be thin and watery, have thick clots, or combine some of both. The blood may be bright red at some points and brownish at others, especially at the beginning and the end of the flow.

When girls get their period they may experience bloating as well as a temporary weight gain. Some girls experience premenstrual tension or Premenstrual Syndrome, which is commonly called PMS. These are changes in hormonal levels that can result in mood swings – so that they feel irritable, angry, weepy and sometimes out of control. It is common for girls in adolescence to have menstrual cramps. Sometimes they are caused by low calcium and magnesium levels. If this is the case, a calcium/magnesium tablet or two along with a glass of milk or cup of hot chocolate with lots of milk may help. Cramps can also be relieved by over-the-counter drugs such as ASA (Aspirin) or Ibuprofen (Advil), as well as by natural and herbal remedies. Some girls suffer from dysmenorrhea, which is the medical term for painful periods. No girl should have to suffer. If the products available don't help make their periods bearable, girls should see their doctor for assessment and for possible prescriptive medication.

Boys and Puberty

While boys can begin puberty as early as nine or as late as sixteen, most of them usually begin puberty at twelve. Puberty may take as few as two and as many as five years. There is no guarantee that if someone has an early start, they will finish early. Sometimes an early starter takes much longer to finish than someone who started late.

The adolescent growth spurt is more intense for boys than it is for girls. Boys grow about 4 inches in the first year of puberty. At the end of puberty, they are about 12 inches taller. Because boys begin puberty later than girls, they have a longer growing period that can continue well into their twenties.

Most of the height that boys gain comes from the lengthening of their torso. While the bones grow longer they don't all grow at the same rate, so that for a while their arms and legs are out of proportion to their trunk. For boys whose legs grow faster than their torso, this period of growth may be one of awkwardness, gawkiness and self-consciousness. Because their feet reach their adult size long before they do, many boys get teased about tripping and about the size of their feet.

Puberty begins with the rapid growth of testes and scrotum. During childhood the scrotum is drawn up close to the body. During puberty it begins to get looser and to hang down. The skin gets darker in color and rougher in texture. The testes and scrotum get larger and the penis gets larger, longer and wider. The age when a boy starts puberty doesn't have anything to do with how large his penis will be when he is fully grown.

Changes also occur in the breasts. The areola may get wider and darker in color and the nipple may also get bigger. Sometimes the breasts feel sore and/or a bump develops under one or both nipples. Sometimes the breasts may swell. This is a reaction to the new hormones and goes away in time. Some boys develop small breasts that spread out and are not noticeable when the rib cage grows to adult size.

Pubic hair begins to appear after the testes have started to develop. The pubic hair first starts to grow at the base of the penis and then on the scrotum. As boys get older, pubic hairs start to grow on the lower belly, down around the anus, and onto the thighs. About a year or so after the pubic hair has started, boys begin to grow hair in their armpits, although for some boys this can start earlier.

For most boys, facial hair begins to appear on the corners of the upper lip when they are between the ages of fourteen and eighteen. It appears earlier for some and later for others. Their sideburns may also start to grow at the same time. Boys don't grow hair on their chin until their genitals are fully developed. As puberty progresses, the hair on their arms and legs gets darker and thicker. Some boys develop hair on their chests and backs while others don't.

Boys are very likely to experience spontaneous erections during puberty. These happen all by themselves without the penis or scrotum being touched or rubbed. As internal changes begin to make boys capable of producing and ejaculating sperm, they begin to have nocturnal emissions or wet dreams. These are the body's way of relieving the testicles of a buildup of sperm through involuntary ejaculations. These ejaculations can happen whether or not boys have masturbated or have had intercourse or erotic dreams. The first ejaculation of semen usually occurs about a year after the beginning of the accelerated penis growth.

As boys reach the latter stages of puberty, their voices begin to change and become lower and deeper. While this process is going on, some boys have a tendency to "crack" or shift suddenly from a low pitch to a high squeaky pitch. This cracking may last for a few months or for as long as a year or two. During this same stage, increased activity causes the sebaceous glands (sweat glands) to secrete a fatty substance causing the skin to break out. Acne is more troublesome in boys than in girls because boys have greater amounts of testosterone.

Boys gain between 50 and 60 pounds during puberty. The male hormone testosterone broadens their shoulders and causes their muscles to grow bigger and stronger than those of girls. The percentage of body weight made up of fat decreases 12-15 percent during puberty, and the percentage of body mass made up of muscle and other lean body tissues increases.[1]

Going through Puberty

For many girls, the experience of puberty sometimes feels as if they've fallen down a kind of "Alice in Wonderland rabbit-hole" and landed in a world where many things appear to be the same but are somehow very, very different. Girls go through so many changes so quickly that their bodies feel new and strange to them. They go to bed at night and wake up in the morning wondering if their jeans are going to fit. They ride the wave of hormones never knowing when they are going to crash. The rules that govern the way they've learned to relate to others are suddenly different, and everyone seems to know this except themselves. People appear to be moving their lips – but it's impossible for girls to understand what's being said.

Even though boys go through a period of awkwardness during puberty where the parts of their bodies don't seem to fit together, and even though they have their own fears and concerns, the developmental dice are still loaded in their favor. When they look in the mirror, the changes that they see are positive and self-affirming. As their bodies get bigger and their shoulders begin to widen, young men embody the very images that we value in males in our society. Parents make a big fuss over their first facial hairs. The first shave is a public celebration of their masculinity. Male sexuality is associated with virility and power. What do Michael Jordan, Ken Griffey Jr., and Eric Lindros have in common? They are big, strong, athletic and make a whole lot of money!

Girls get the short end of the stick. They find themselves in a double bind as they enter puberty. Along with their newly developed bodies comes the pressure to look good and to fit into a narrowly defined ideal of female beauty. The same fat that biology considers necessary for female sexuality is not acceptable in what is considered the ideal female. Instead of celebrating their rounded bodies, most girls feel conflicted over how they experience themselves and how society is telling them they should be. They begin to feel as if their bodies are out of control as they gain weight. Because there is no place in our society for girls to talk about their feelings over their changing bodies and because no one celebrates the changes that are taking place, many girls encode their feelings in the language of fat. They deal with their discomfort by feeling fat. They try to control the changing shape of their bodies and the subsequent changes in their lives by dieting.

> "Ever since Sarah began puberty," laments her mother, Trisha, "she is always telling me that she is so fat. I want to tell her that if she is so concerned with her weight, all she has to do is stop snacking. But I'm afraid to say anything to her because I don't want to make an issue of food."

When girls feel fat during puberty they are not talking about their weight. Helping them to change their eating habits makes them feel frustrated and misunderstood because it doesn't address the real issues that lie underneath.

The Pressure of Maturing Too Early, the Pain of Maturing Too Late

Girls don't all begin puberty at the same time. There may be girls in their class who have already finished puberty at ten or eleven, and girls who have yet to begin. For girls at either end of the developmental continuum, puberty can be more difficult because they stand out. Girls who mature early look different and are self-conscious. Because they look like adults, people sometimes expect adult behavior from them at a time when emotionally and cognitively they are still children. Boys and men relate to them in a more sexualized way because their bodies look sexually mature. Instead of feeling excited about their changing bodies, they feel embarrassment and shame.

> "Sarah doesn't want us to see that the attention boys pay to her body bothers her," continues Trisha. "She's got good comebacks. She's not going to be cowed by it or anything. She does seem to be aware that boys might be attracted to her just because she is developed. We've tried to tell her that being noticed because you have breasts is not a good reason to have all the attention."

Often girls deal with their discomfort by feeling fat and by encoding their feelings in the language of fat. When we encourage girls to look at what lies underneath they often talk about the pain of being different. They talk about what it's like to be teased. They talk about the changes in their lives.

"The other kids tease me, says eleven-year-old Alison. "They call me a mute [mutation]. At recess the boys try to grab my breasts. I get really angry at them."

Her friend Jennie laments, "My mother thinks that just because I got my period all I'm going to be interested in is boys. She keeps wanting to know about everything that I am doing ... I'm not allowed to hang out with my friends as much. I guess I'd like to tell her that she's really unfair."

Girls who mature early sometimes begin to date prematurely, and then run the risk of being pressured to become sexually active when they are not ready.

"My boyfriend is sixteen," says thirteen-year-old Tiffany. "I like kissing him, but he keeps bugging me to, um, you know, to have sex. I'm afraid that if I say no he'll think that I don't love him and he'll go find someone else."

Girls who mature later than their friends also have to deal with being out of step with everyone else.

"The kids in school always tease me," says twelve-year-old Clare. "They yell: 'Clare, Clare, no pubic hair. Her front looks the same as her back.'"

Twelve-year-old Jane says, "Last year I was really good friends with these girls. Now they all have their period. They call me 'baby' and won't let me hang out with them."

"Everyone seems to have their period except me," says twelve-year-old Rachel. "I really want it so I don't feel so left out. My mom got hers when she was almost thirteen. Does that mean I will get mine soon?"

Thirteen-year-old Patty talks about how alone she feels. She says, "About a year ago my mom bought me a padded bra because I wasn't growing in my chest area. The first day I wore it everybody noticed that my boobs seemed to be bigger. They thought I had stuffed my bra. I told one girl because she was bugging me so much and she told everyone else. People started to whisper and were asking me why I wear a padded bra. I had to lie and say I didn't but they still make fun of me."

Girls also go through a developmental period during adolescence when they are egocentric or quite preoccupied with themselves. They think that they are the only ones to have these feelings and fears. They also believe that what is happening to them at this moment will continue to happen to them forever. It's no wonder that their angst is magnified and their feelings are so intense.

We can't make things better for girls even if we want to. We can't solve their problems no matter how hard we try. What we can do is listen responsively and validate their feelings. We can say things like "That sounds terrible. I know how awful it must be to feel different and to be teased." We can share our own experiences of puberty with girls so they know that they are not alone in what they feel, or even worse, that something terrible is happening to them. We can let them know that they will not feel this way forever. They need to know that everything evens out as they get older, and that eventually their bodies settle down.

Getting Your Period

Although their first period is a major event in girls' lives, it very rarely receives any acknowledgment or attention. How many families do you know that announce at the dinner table that Sally just got her first period? How many girls do you know who rush into their sixth, seventh or eighth grade class joyously proclaiming that they have begun to bleed?

Most of us have internalized centuries of societal taboos around menstruation – despite the fact that we consider ourselves modern and liberated women. We ourselves sometimes can't help seeing the girls and women who menstruate or the process of menstruation itself as "unclean." Look at how we talk about it: we have "the curse," or our "monthly." It's "that time of the month" for women who are "on the rag." Have you ever noticed that the word *blood* never passes our lips? Even though tampons and sanitary napkins have now made it into the popular culture, we also never hear the word *blood* mentioned on TV. Every time I see the commercials I wonder how many girls and women think that when they have their period it *should* be blue!?

Many of us women have trouble talking about our bodies. Many of our mothers passed their own discomfort and shame on to us because they were uncomfortable with theirs.

> Cheryl teaches seventh grade girls. She says, "I remember when I was eleven. My mother gave me a booklet called *How to Tell My Daughter*. It was put out by Modess. She just sort of threw it at me and told me to read it and ask her if I had any questions. She disappeared so quickly that I knew there was no way in hell that I would ever take the risk of asking her anything that was important to me."

> "I knew that girls got their periods and stuff like that," says Jean, the mother of eleven-year-old Fiona. "We had this film at school and they gave you this nice book. I thought, 'I want my hair to be like this woman on the book.' But you know, everything is so clean in the book and when you get your period, you feel dirty. You feel sweaty. You have to constantly change your pad. When I didn't have my period I was so thrilled."

> "I remember that film," Louise exclaims. "I got pretty excited about it thinking about how the body works and I

came rushing home. My mother was gardening out in the back and I said, 'Mom, guess what! We had a film on menstruation.' And she went, 'Shush. You know, that's not something that you talk about.' Well right there and then I got a clear message that that was something that should go underground."

We learn to be very private and even secretive about our periods. We hide our tampons and sanitary pads underneath the bathroom sink. Can you imagine what would happen if we went public? Imagine standing up in a meeting and telling everyone that you have to go and change your pad! And somewhere out there I'm sure that there must be a cosmic rule that says the first time we get our periods, we are usually wearing white.

"I remember," says Sonia, the mother of eleven-year-old Carla, "that for years and years I kept seeing my mother keep her own pads and everything in a locked drawer, and asking her repeatedly what was in there. She would tell me, 'I'll tell you when you are older.' Finally, one day I guess when I was about ten or eleven she did finally tell me what this was for."

When girls get their first period, it usually comes without warning. Instead of celebrating a natural transition, most girls are self-conscious and embarrassed. They are mortified if anyone else finds out – especially the boys.

Says twelve-year-old Moira, "The boys tease us about our periods. They tell us that our pads are showing and that we smell like fish."

Girls have a lot of questions about their periods and about their changing bodies. Whenever I brought books about puberty into grade seven groups, the girls were eager to read them. It only took a little bit of encouragement for them to talk about their concerns.

"I noticed that I have started to grow in my chest," said Emily. "Does this have anything to do with your periods?"

"My breasts hurt sometimes," said Vanessa. "Does this mean that I have cancer?"

"How will I know when it will come?" asked Megan. "And will it hurt?"

"What happens if I get it in the middle of class?" Clare wanted to know.

"The first time I had my period," Jing said, "the blood didn't look like real blood. Did that mean that there was something wrong with me?"

"If I don't get my period every month, does that mean that I'm not normal?" asked Michelle.

"Am I always going to gain weight around my period?" asked Carita.

"What does *anemia* mean?" asked Helene. "Am I going to get anemia?"

"Why do girls get nervous when they get their periods?" asked Alana.

"Sometimes when I get my period," shared Maria, "I feel as if there is a huge pressure building up inside my head. My ears get blocked and I can't hear anything that anybody is saying. My friends can't see that there is anything wrong because I'm so quiet but inside I think that I am going to burst with anger."

Many times girls don't get the chance to ask the questions that are most important to them or to really learn about how their bodies work. In her book, *The "What's Happening to My Body?" Book for Girls*, Lynda Madaras states that "elementary school children including seventh-graders don't need sex education, they need puberty education. Kids of this age have a multitude of questions and fears about the changes that are or soon will be taking place in their bodies. These children need reassuring puberty education before they are ready for sex education."

"When Bonnie got her period," says her mother Jessica, "she knew what it was, not like me. I thought I had the runs. I had no idea of what it was like. And we celebrated. We bought her a rose and we said welcome to the club of women. Her music teacher gave her a journal. She was quite pleased that we made a big deal of it."

We need to let girls know that their bodies and the changes in their bodies are normal, healthy and natural. We have to help girls celebrate their bodies instead of feeling ashamed of them. We also need to provide them with information when they ask for it, and be willing to listen to their concerns.

"I would really like my daughter to learn about her body," says Sue.

"I wish that I had been talked to about puberty in a particular way that wouldn't have made it such a big deal, and that respected me. I would have liked people to talk to me as a person and not as a kid," concludes Jean.

Time Out for Yourself

- What was your own puberty like? Where did you fit on the continuum – did you develop early, late or in the middle with the rest of the girls?

- How similar was your development to that of your daughter? How was it different?

- How did you learn about puberty, menstruation and the changes in your body?

- What would you have wanted to know?

- What kind of information would you like your daughter to have?

- How comfortable are you talking about puberty and menstruation with your daughter?

- What kind of information, support or resources would you need to make you more comfortable, or to ensure that she receives the kind of information that you would want her to have?

- How comfortable are you with your daughter's changing body? What makes you feel uncomfortable? How do you handle your discomfort?

- Are you more strict with your daughter now that her body is changing?

Time with Each Other

- **Share yourself.** You don't have to be a perfect mother (or aunt, teacher, nurse, etc.) to be able to talk to girls about their bodies. You don't have to be totally "together," or completely self-assured, or be able to whip out the perfect talk for the perfectly appropriate moment. It's all right not to know everything, to be self-conscious, or unsure, or even a little bit embarrassed or uncomfortable. We carry our own histories with us, which is part of what makes us unique. They are also part of what makes it difficult for us to talk about things like masturbation, intercourse or being attracted to someone of the same sex. Girls don't need us to be technical experts. What they do need is for us to be honest and to be ourselves. When we admit to being uncomfortable, we give them permission for their own discomfort. When we share our own experiences, we open the door for girls to share their concerns with us.

- **Initiate the conversation.** In the next section, I'll go into more detail about *The Talk*. For now, I want to suggest that it's up to you to initiate the conversations about puberty. Just telling girls that they can ask us questions almost guarantees that they never will. Girls need to know how sincere we are in our offer. The best way to invite their confidences is to begin by sharing some of our own.

- **Share the resources.** There are a number of good books about puberty. I've listed some in the final section of this book under Resources. I learned a lot of things about puberty and about my own body that I never knew before when I read these books. You can read them together with your girl if both of you feel comfortable doing so. You can also leave the books around and suggest that she mark off the topics or pages that she would like you to read.

- **Keep a growth chart or a journal.** Some of the books about puberty contain a growth chart that girls can use, or you can make your own. Keeping a chart (or a journal) allows girls to record, acknowledge and become more comfortable with the changes in their bodies. It's important to respect girls' privacy. We need to let them know that their journals belong to them and that they don't need to share the details of every pubic hair that they discover.

- **Dig out the old photographs.** Photographs are a wonderful way of giving girls a *context* – letting them know that other people have had the same experiences. If you have photographs of yourself growing up, or of the other women in your family, use them as a way of looking at the changes that you have all gone through.

- **Reclaim the tampons and sanitary napkins.** Take them out from under the sink and make a public declaration of your femininity. Put them in a basket, tie a ribbon around the basket and put it on the counter in the bathroom. You can both giggle together about some of the comments you will receive.

- **Celebrate her first period.** Make a big deal of it. Bake her a cake or buy her a rose. It is something to celebrate!

NOTES

1   The information on puberty has been taken from the following books:

Diane F. Paplia and Sally Wendkos Olds. *A Child's World: Infancy through Adolescence.* New York: McGraw Hill, 1990.

Laurence Steinberg and Jay Belsky. *Infancy, Childhood & Adolescence: Development in Context.* New York: McGraw Hill, 1991.

Lynda Madaras. *The "What's Happening to My Body?" Book for Girls.* New York: Newmarket Press, 1988.

10

Sexuality

Girls begin to develop "crushes" around sixth grade. Crushes are safe because they are acted out from a distance. Girls develop crushes on rock stars and movie stars. Some girls develop crushes on older girls. The first crushes that girls have on boys have more to do with speculation than with interaction. They are almost like a trial run, a sort of dress rehearsal for the real thing. Given the chance, girls will spend hours talking about which boys they like, which boys their friends like, and whether or not the boys like them in return. Girls tease each other and tease the boys mercilessly. Their interactions are fraught with titillation, excitement and sometimes even hurt. The secret shared with a friend one day becomes common knowledge the next as confidences are broken and "secrets" are spread around the school. Girls are both victims and victimizers. The girl who feels hurt today can usually be found teasing someone else tomorrow.

"I listen to Lucy and her friends talking," says her mom, Sheila. "One of them will talk about a specific boy and ask the others, 'Do you think he likes me?' and then her friend will call the boy and ask him 'Do you like Lucy, or do you like Jennie?' They put each other into such terrible situations."

Giggles, tears and the intensity that goes along with them are part of the process that transforms boys and girls from the kids who sit next to each other in kindergarten to potential heterosexual mates. As girls begin to see boys differently, they also begin to change.

"There are these two girls in my class," says Jessica. "They wear really short shorts and makeup. They talk about going to dances and things. They kind of brag about it. One girl was bragging about the cologne that this boy was wearing. It was like she was dancing with this boy and the next morning she could still smell his cologne he was wearing so much."

Not all girls become interested in boys at the same time. Nor do all girls become interested in boys. Some girls are aware of their attraction to other girls at an early age, but are rarely encouraged to talk about these feelings. Like late bloomers, not fitting into the mainstream is difficult for them. Many girls often turn their feelings against themselves and feel fat. When girls are able to decode the language of fat, they can talk about how they really feel.

Says Emily: "The girls in my class, all they ever do is hang out and talk about boys and other stuff that doesn't interest me. Sometimes I feel really lonely – like I'll never have friends."

By seventh grade, girls and boys begin to experiment with hold-ing hands and kissing. They want to know what to do when their hands are sweaty.[1] They worry about not knowing how to kiss. They talk about open-mouth kissing and about the "popular" girls – girls with breasts who belong to the "make-out" group in the school.

> Says twelve-year-old Brandy: "Megan and Susie and I went to this party at Lara's house on the weekend. We started to play *truth or dare* and Stephen dared me to kiss Ryan. I just closed my eyes and hoped for the best."

> According to twelve-year-old Michelle, "We're not sup-posed to kiss or anything like that in our school, but kids go outside and do it anyway. I told Sean that I liked him and wanted to kiss him. He told me to meet him by the park-ing lot but then he didn't show up."

Girls in seventh grade are intensely curious about sex and about the intricacies of relationships.

> "Bonnie came up to me one day," says her mom, Jessica, "and asked me what happens to the ugly boys. She wanted to know if they ever have sex. 'Well,' I said, 'remember I told you before that you see couples and sometimes the woman is really pretty and the man is really ugly or the man is really handsome and the woman isn't but, you know, they see something beautiful in each other and so they're not ugly to each other.'"

In one seventh grade class that I visited, the teacher told the girls that I was there to talk about "family life education." It took me a while to realize that she was talking about sex. While I could "talk the talk" I realized how uncomfortable I was when the time came to "walk the walk." I didn't know how much to tell the girls.

I wasn't sure what the policy concerning sex education was in this particular school and community. But because I didn't want to disappoint the girls, I told them that I would answer their questions the next week if they wrote them out and gave them to me at the end of the class. Here are some of the things that girls worry about:[2]

- Where do twins come from?

- What is masturbation? How do you masturbate?

- What is a blow job? How do you do it?

- How do gay people have sex?

- When is a safe time to have sex?

- Can you have sex when you have your period?

- What is herpes?

- Should I practice *safe sex* using a condom on a carrot or wiener if I am planning on having sex? Is that what *practicing* safe sex means?

- I have a friend who had sex at a young age and somehow the word got around. She now is being called a slut. Is she a slut?

- Should you have sex to feel loved?

- I have a friend whose other friend's older brother is bugging her and trying to talk her into having sex with him. What should she do?

- My friend is twelve but really wants to have sex. She talks about it a lot and always thinks of it. Is that wrong?

- I have a very good friend who has had sex three times and twice the condom broke. She has missed her period once and is very worried. Can you give her any advice?

- I have a friend who lately has been looking down my shirt, staring at my chest and "accidentally" touching me. I'm afraid she is a lesbian. What should I do?

Our Attitudes toward Sex

Girls and boys have different attitudes toward sex and experience their sexuality differently. Boys experience themselves as sexual beings with their first erections and wet dreams even if these are spontaneous and have little to do with sex. Most boys have their first sexual experiences early in adolescence, which usually occur through masturbation. They experience sexual satisfaction that has nothing to do with intimacy. The first time that many adolescent boys have intercourse, the same separation between sex and intimacy exists.

Often when boys describe their first time to their male friends, they get their overwhelming approval.[3] Because of the hierarchical nature of boys' relationships – and because boys get their self-esteem from what they do – a boy's first and subsequent experiences of intercourse have little to do with intimacy and more to do with achievement, with "scoring." Boys learn that they are players in the game of sexuality. They are studs. Each time that they score validates their masculinity. It is usually only when they get older that young men learn to integrate emotional intimacy into their sexual relationships.

When girls learn about their bodies it is usually in terms of menstruation and reproduction. The first time that girls get their periods, their thoughts aren't likely to be about sex. Girls learn about ovaries and uteruses. They are warned about the risks of pregnancy. They are told that it is their job to keep male sexuality in check. Very rarely do girls learn about orgasms, sexual pleasure, or about making choices other than saying "no."

A girl's first sexual encounter is often with a boy that she feels close to.[4] The first time she has intercourse it is most likely with someone she feels she is in love with. Girls don't talk about their first sexual experiences as easily as boys do. When they do share their experiences with their female friends, they receive a mixed reaction. Sometimes they are even met with disapproval – because girls who act on their sexuality run the risk of being labeled as sluts.[5] Girls know about and worry about this double standard even before they are ready to have sex.

"I don't like it when girls are thought of as sluts and guys are rewarded," says Morgan. "What I mean by that is if a girl has sex with a guy and they aren't a couple she is told she is a slut or 'trash.' When a guy has sex with a girl and they aren't going out together, he is slapped on the back and told he has accomplished something good. First of all, it is no one else's business who, when, and why a girl sleeps with someone. Second of all, why are girls labeled like that and guys not? For example, you don't go up to a guy who has been having sex with a different girl every week and say 'You're a slut.' That just doesn't happen."

"I think what this all comes down to is how men and women are treated differently. Girls have to be loyal and faithful, and guys are allowed to be whatever they want. I'm not saying all guys are like this and that all girls are called sluts, but it still happens. I disagree with the term "slut" and maybe if more people minded their own business it wouldn't be used."

While many boys have sex, many girls have love. They believe that sex is something that happens in the heat of passion. The first time that girls have intercourse, most of them don't use any form of contraception. Many believe that they can't become pregnant the first time. Girls believe that romantic sex is spontaneous sex. If you have a condom on hand it means that you planned to have sex – something that makes you look like a slut. Many teenage girls have unprotected sex because they are afraid that they will lose the boy's love if they ask him to use condoms. Some girls are afraid to assert themselves because they are afraid of the boy's disapproval. Some girls say they feel that they don't know the boy well enough.

Giving Girls Information

Girls today are having sex at younger and younger ages. The number of girls who begin to have intercourse at the age of fifteen has risen dramatically in the past ten years.[6] When girls don't have the knowledge or skills with which to practice safe sex, they leave themselves open to pregnancy and also to sexually transmitted diseases (STDs). Genital herpes and yeast infections cause discomfort. Chlamydia can seriously affect the reproductive organs and leave girls sterile. AIDS can kill them. We still have a myth that only gay men can get AIDS – even though the rising numbers of cases among heterosexual women prove otherwise. The chances of contracting AIDS through heterosexual contact is sixteen times greater for females than for males. Adolescent girls and young women are the fastest growing group of people contracting HIV infection. No matter how nice or wonderful the boy is, or how good a family he comes from, character references and instinct are still not as important or effective as the use of a condom.

Girls need to receive information about their bodies and their sexuality so they can take charge of their lives. It is sometimes difficult for us to provide girls with the kind of information that they need because most of us have grown up with shame. Girls take our silence and discomfort as a profound message that anything to do with their bodies and with sex is taboo – a subject that will get them into trouble when they speak. When they can't ask us questions, they turn to the misinformation that comes from their friends.

Sex education that is offered in the school system seldom tells girls what they really need to know because school boards walk a tightrope between balancing the moral and religious needs of parents with ensuring quality sexual health. Sometimes parents object to the schools offering what they see as something that is the total responsibility of the family. Sometimes people feel that if you give children information about sex, you're just encouraging them to be sexually active.

Sex education does not cause children to become sexually active. Studies show that the countries with the lowest rates of teenage pregnancy and childbirth have the most liberal attitudes about sex. They show that children whose parents teach them about birth control will practice contraception at a far greater rate than those whose parents say nothing. Those areas in North America where the only form of contraception that kids learn is "just say no to sex" have the highest rates in the developed world for teen pregnancy, abortions and births.[7]

Most of us share the concern that girls will have sex when they are not emotionally ready for it, or because they are pressured into it by their peers. We try to deal with this concern by believing that we have the power to stop them by telling them it isn't right. Yet as girls approach adolescence other competing influences stake their claim. Friends become a powerful authority, while messages from the popular culture sexualize girls earlier and earlier in their lives.

As girls grow older, they take offense at the very idea that they can be pressured into something. No one likes to be told that they are influenced by other people. When we see it happening, we have to find a way of addressing it that doesn't make girls feel put down or condescended to. When I spoke to an auditorium of high school students about how hard it is for girls to say no, several angry girls confronted me afterward. They reacted to my speaking in what they felt were generalizations, especially in front of the boys. "Girls also get horny," they told me. "Nobody pushes us around or tells us what to do. We make the decisions to have sex." In the rush to make girls equal to boys, we have to make sure that girls' sexuality doesn't become just a replica of the boys', but is an integrated part of who the girls are.

Talking to Girls about Sex

Many of us have grown up with *The Talk*. It usually took place during puberty when we were just about to get our periods. As our mothers told us the facts of life, it was never really clear who felt more uncomfortable and who would succeed in getting out of the room first. Those of us who came from more sexually liberated households might have been spared some of the discomfort, but we still didn't learn what we really wanted to know. Despite our parents' best intentions most of them had difficulty with our budding sexuality because they were uncomfortable with their own. Today, many of us are still dealing with our own embarrassment – so it's hard for us not to emulate our mothers and give girls our own variation of *The Talk*. Although we may want to be more open, we're still not sure of how to go about talking about puberty or sex in a more personalized way.

According to Meg Hickling, author of *Speaking of SEX*, the best time to give girls information about puberty and about sex is when the questions begin to come. This means teaching girls about their bodies when they are very young. Hickling also suggests that we give girls information about the changes in their bodies before the changes begin to take place.[8] Sex education (or puberty education) is a lot more than a one-time-only talk about the facts of life. It's an ongoing dialogue. It's an opportunity to impart not only information but also values, to exchange confidences, to disclose fears and to explore what it means to be a girl and woman today.

Girls are eager for information and have many concerns. They also feel really vulnerable about their changing bodies and their sexuality. If these have not been hot topics in your household before, girls will rarely break what they perceive as a taboo by initiating conversations. Sometimes it takes them quite some time to feel safe enough to respond to your own attempts. Regardless of how good your intentions are now, they might be met by silence or bravado. Even though you might want to talk, they might feel that it is not cool to ask questions. By seventh grade, girls often feel that they have to appear as if they already know it all.

> "When Brandy was younger she was very curious and we did answer to the best that we could in anything that she asked, but now she doesn't ask us. I have tried to take the opportunity to talk to her when we are in the car, but she threatens to get out. She listens to me but it's only under duress."

> "There are things that I would have liked to know about sex," says Sheila. "I'm not telling them to Lucy. I guess I'm waiting for her to come and ask me, and I don't think that she will."

"I would really like my daughter to know about her body," Jessica says. "But when I try to bring it up, Bonnie says, 'I know this stuff. I've been kissed. I know how to kiss open-mouth.'"

Instead of sitting girls down for *The Talk*, it helps to prepare the ground for open communication by spending time alone together – not just talking about puberty and sexuality, but also about the other issues in our lives. Carly and her daughter Kate have regular "Mother-to-Daughter" sessions.

"When Kate tells me that she needs a Mother-to-Daughter, I know that something is bothering her – something that she wants to talk to me about. I make sure that we have time alone just for the two of us."

Sometimes the best sharing comes not from a planned discussion but when we are doing things informally with each other. It helps to do dishes together, bake a cake, take a walk. We can introduce the topics into activities that we are doing in a casual way, and share our experiences with girls without requiring any response from them in return. We can say things like, "I remember when my breasts began to grow. I felt really weird" or "I remember when the other girls started to get their periods and I really wanted mine" (or had it first, or worried that it wouldn't come). In chapter 9 on puberty I talked about how we don't need to be perfect, and how it is all right to be embarrassed, as long as we share our embarrassment with the girls.

When we start to share our experiences with girls, we sometimes have trouble knowing what information to give and what information to hold back. We want them to know everything – but we are a little queasy when it comes to sharing things that we considered personal up until now. It's important for us to recognize that there are boundaries. We selectively share ourselves to create equality and, thus, intimacy between us so that girls will feel safe in talking about their concerns. We have to recognize, however, that no matter how open we are or how much we care about girls, they are not our best friends and are not entitled to confidences that we would only share with our partners or with our peers.

"Melanie is not my best friend," says Pat. "There are many things that I can't share with her, and there will be things that she won't want to share with me. I like it that way."

"Jessica is coming to the age when she wants to deal with sexuality and, because I have no guide from my family, I have to sort of wing it. The other day she asked me if I have ever done oral sex and I thought, 'Oh God what do I say now?' And I said, 'You know, a person's sexual activity or what they do with other people is really private. If you want to know what oral sex is, I'd be happy to tell you about it but I don't feel comfortable talking about my experiences.'"

If we can be open with girls about sexuality, we can give them the opportunity to talk about the different messages they receive, and to evaluate what these messages mean to them. We can address their concerns as they arise.

"Zoe told me one day that she was horny," said Rena. "I said to her, 'Why don't you masturbate?' She was horrified. I said to her, 'People don't always have or need a sexual partner, you know.' She hates when I talk about masturbation. It takes away her fantasy of true love."

"Fiona said to me, 'I think I'm ready to have sex.' I tried not to choke and said to her, 'Well, this is a stage that your body is going through. You're having all these feelings. This is a time when you have to learn what these feelings are and what they mean.' It turned out that she was going to a party and was afraid that she wouldn't know how to kiss."

If girls feel that we are free of judgment, then they feel free to talk about their fears. If we can recognize and validate that desire, we can give them alternatives other than intercourse with which to explore their sexuality. We can help girls integrate their sexuality into their lives and make healthy choices for themselves.

 ## Time Out for Yourself

- How did you learn about sex and sexuality?

- What would you have wanted to know?

- What kind of information would you like your daughter to have?

- How comfortable do you feel talking to her?

- What resources are available to you?

- Who do you think should tell her about sex?

- How much do you think she should know?

- How do you feel about sex education in your school?

- How do you feel about teaching her about safe sex?

- How old would you like her to be when she first has sex? In what circumstances should this be?

- How do you impart your values and beliefs to your daughter? How much room is there for discussion and disagreement?

NOTES

1 Dr. Carol J. Eagle and Carol Colman. *All That She Can Be: Helping Your Daughter Achieve Her Full Potential and Maintain Her Self-Esteem during the Critical Years of Adolescence*. New York: Simon and Schuster, 1993, pp. 171, 172, 179.

2 Thanks to Carly McFetridge, community health nurse with the Vancouver Health Board, for her additions to this list.

3 Laurence Steinberg and Jay Belsky. *Infancy, Childhood and Adolescence: Development in Context*. New York: McGraw Hill, 1991, pp. 483-484.

4 Steinberg and Belsky.

5 Steinberg and Belsky.

6 Eagle and Colman.

7 William A. Fisher, Donna Bryne and Leonard A. White. "Emotional Barriers to Contraception" in *Adolescents, Sex and Contraception*. Hillsdale, NJ: Lawrence Erlbaum, 1983, p. 234.

8 Meg Hickling. *Speaking of SEX: Are You Ready to Answer the Questions Your Kids Will Ask?* Kelowna, BC: Northstone Publishing, 1996, pp. 57-58.

11

Food

It used to be that when someone said they had been "bad" the night before, we knew that we were talking about sex. And from the tone of their voice, which often bordered on the verge of bragging, we knew that whatever they had done, they were somewhat proud of it. Today, when someone says that they have been "bad" we take it for granted that whatever they have done has to do with food. It could have been a major binge. It could have been eating just one piece of cake for dessert. It could even have been having a normal meal. Whatever it was, its aftermath certainly includes shame – for wanting, for eating and for enjoying what they ate.

As women, most of us grow up into an uneasy relationship with food and with eating. We learn to categorize what we eat into foods that we really want but can't have, foods we should have but don't want, foods we think are healthy and foods we think will make us fat. We are supposed to do the cooking, but we're not supposed to eat. If we allow ourselves to eat with gusto and without apology, we're seen as aggressive and unfeminine. We learn to pick at our food in public and overeat in secret. We rarely approach food with joy, but instead are consumed by deprivation and guilt. No matter how diligently we try to reduce the fat we eat, we can't get the siren call of Oreo cookies out of our head.

When I first read Marissa Piesman's mystery novel *Heading Uptown*, I laughed with recognition as her character Nina Fishman described our erratic relationship with food:

> Nina worried about the excessive consumption of sweets by so many women. It had a misguided decadent edge to it, up there with women in high heels and men without socks. Not that she had a right to be self-righteous about any kind of food craziness, considering the weird shit she'd consumed over the years. She really had no right to be judgmental. But Nina saw this socially acceptable practice of skipping the entree and heading straight for dessert in political terms. Real women ate real food. To pretend that you could exist solely on imported chocolate or the pastry basket at Bruce's was to deny that you were a human being who needed to be fueled up periodically.[1]

Most of us don't eat real food. We often don't know when we're actually hungry and have difficulty figuring out when we're full. Our knowledge of nutrition comes mainly from counting calories and grams of fat, so we rarely think in terms of fueling our bodies or of making ourselves strong.

We pass on our own attitudes, beliefs, and our ambivalence toward food to the girls in our lives. At dinner at a friend's house, I listened to a six-year-old explain how she could only eat one piece of bread because she was afraid of getting fat. In a classroom discussion with sixth grade students, an eleven-year-old girl described how her family counted everybody's calories and restricted their grams of fat.

"My mother says that if I start watching what I eat now, I won't gain weight later on," she said, "and I'll even get to live two years longer when I grow up."

While our unresolved relationships with food do not in themselves create eating disorders, they can strengthen an existing preoccupation with food and weight. If we are going to help girls accept that real women and real girls need real food, we must first begin by examining our own beliefs and attitudes so that we can understand what we are passing on to the girls in our lives. The following questions might help you sort out how you think and feel.

---

e x a m i n i n g   **your attitudes toward food**

How often do you:
- Divide foods into "good" foods and "bad" foods?
- Let yourself eat "forbidden" foods?
- Let yourself eat "forbidden" foods in public?
- Eat in secret?
- Talk about diets, calories and fat grams?
- Forbid "junk" food from being in your house?
- Feel guilty when you eat dessert?
- Count fat grams or calories?
- Use words like "pigging out"?
- Qualify your eating with "I shouldn't have this, but ...?

If you answered *frequently* or *a lot* to many of the questions, ask yourself how often you sit down and eat a balanced meal. When you examine your own attitudes toward food, it's important to remember that you don't have to be perfect or make drastic changes in the way that you eat. Most of us have an erratic relationship with food. We are the products of the same culture as the girls in our lives. It's much more helpful for girls if we are willing to admit to and share our own struggles with our relationship with food – and thus open a door for girls to share theirs.

The Different Meanings of Food

Our relationship to food goes far beyond just fueling our bodies and keeping us strong. Food has many meanings for us. It has an impact on many areas of our lives. Food is social. We congregate around the kitchen table, share our problems over coffee, have friends in for dinner, and blow out the candles on our birthday cakes. Preparing food can be an act of nurturing. Sometimes we cook and bake and feed others as a way of showing our love. Many of our cultural traditions and religious traditions are centered around food. We have special foods for Thanksgiving, Christmas, Passover, Diwali and Chinese New Year. We break the Muslim fast of Ramadan. Many of us reach for the chicken soup whenever we have a cold.

Our relationship with food also has a dark side. For some of us, family meals and holiday occasions were battlefields where scores were settled, and criticism and blame were meted out. Traditionally, food is served in its best and largest proportions to the men in our society. In many cultures, women and girls are given less to eat and the food that they do receive is less nutritious and of poorer quality. In areas of the world where there is famine, women and girls are at the end of the line. Having a smaller portion used to be seen as ladylike and dainty – remember Scarlett O'Hara? She picked at her food like a bird in public and then ate like a real person in the privacy of her room. Fanatical Christian girls were praised in years gone by for refusing to eat, fainting, and having hallucinations (visions from the Lord). Their wasted bodies were seen as proof that they could live on faith alone.[2]

In many North American families, women are responsible for all the cooking and serving. They tend to eat last, and sometimes end up with left-overs, while men receive their meals hot and get the first helpings of a dish. Girls growing up learn that no matter who Mom may be in the outside world, at home she is the one who gets the broken piece of the pie.

Girls and Food

Even if girls are picky eaters as children, we still see a shift as their relationship with food begins to change in adolescence. By the latter part of sixth grade, girls begin to skip breakfast. They talk about not being hungry in the morning. Sometimes there is no food in the house. Sometimes there is no one home or awake to prepare it, or to talk to while they are eating. Some girls are responsible for younger children (either their siblings or their neighbor's children), and have no time to eat themselves. Regardless of the reasons why girls don't eat, the results are the same. At some point in the morning, they begin to feel tired and to feel "spaced out." They start to see themselves as stupid because they can't make the connection between running on empty and not being able to perform in class.

Girls internalize society's attitudes toward food. During puberty they are faced with the conflict between their fear of getting fat and the needs of their growing bodies, which make them hungry all the time.

> "I eat and eat and think that I'm not normal," says Jenna. "My mother says that I'm going through a growth spurt, but I'm afraid of getting fat."

> "How much food should I eat?" asks Zoe. "Do I have to eat vegetables every day?"

Like Nina Fishman, many girls will opt for sugar instead of real food. In one grade seven group, the girls used to come to the meetings by way of the grocery store. They would arrive laden down with enough sugar foods to support the economy of a small Caribbean island. In another grade eight group, the girls would detour via the school cafeteria where they would stock up on the specialty of raw cookie dough. While our teeth ached watching them, we never made a direct issue of their choices – because we recognized the context in which they were made.

Junk food and its counterpart (healthy and nutritious food) take on particular meanings in adolescence. They become a vital part of the peer culture and reflect the developmental tasks and conflicts that girls struggle with at this time. According to Dr. Gwen Chapman, girls choose junk foods because they taste good, because they are convenient and because they are affordable. Junk foods are associated with pleasure and with friends and with snacking. Eating junk foods is a way for girls to assert their independence and develop ties with their peers. However, due to society's preoccupation with thinness, junk foods also have negative connotations – going off a diet, being out of control, overeating and feeling guilty.

Some girls associate healthy foods with family meals and with being at home. Eating family food is one way to remain connected to their families whom most girls acknowledge as being important to them. Girls see healthy foods as being "good for you" because they are high in nutritious value, and they don't contain "bad" substances such as fat, sugar, cholesterol and preservatives. These foods are associated with being on a diet, being good and being in control.[3]

During adolescence, girls are constantly engaged in a balancing act: they want to be independent and remain attached to important family ties. They want to be thin and yet also satisfy their cravings for sugar and fat. Many of them deal with this dilemma through their use of food. They alternate between "pigging out" and feeling guilty, and dieting and feeling in control. The erratic eating pattern that girls learn in adolescence can play havoc with their health further down the road.

Girls and Nutrition

We often smile indulgently at the "growing" boy and urge him to eat, regardless of how much he weighs. We want him to become big and strong and fit into our image of the ideal man. When we look at the "growing" girl, we tend to become uneasy when we calculate how much she consumes. We try to restrict her food intake because we are afraid she is going to get fat. This can have a negative effect on girls because the amount they eat and the nutrients they receive have to be related to the stage of puberty they are in. Instead of reducing their fat intake and depriving them of fuel and energy when they are growing, it's far better for us to teach girls how to achieve a balance in the food that they eat, and to encourage them to use their bodies and to be active.

We also need to look at the kinds of foods that girls eat once they have finished puberty. Studies show that teenage girls in North America eat too much fat and protein and salt, not enough carbohydrates, and less than the Recommended Nutrient Intake (RNI) or Recommended Dietary Allowance (RDA) for some micronutrients – especially iron and calcium and zinc.[4] Girls need iron to replace the amount lost during menstruation and to avoid the risk of anemia. Calcium is important for skeletal growth and for building bone density in order to prevent osteoporosis down the road. Zinc is needed for growth and for sexual maturation.

Because so much of our knowledge of food is linked to diets and to our fear of getting fat, most of us don't know the role that different foods play in our bodies or how to achieve balance in our lives. We also don't know how much direction to give girls. We want them to eat for health and enjoyment but are afraid if we make an issue of it they will become overly preoccupied with food. I have provided some guidelines for you and your family. Remember that the goal of healthy eating is to achieve a balance. This means that eating chocolate and going to McDonald's are still things you can enjoy.

Strategies to Consider

- Enjoy a good variety of foods.
- Emphasize cereals, breads and other grain products, vegetables and fruits.
- Choose lower-fat dairy products, leaner meats and food prepared with little or no fats.

- Limit your intake of salt, alcohol and caffeine.

- Avoid terms like "healthy eating" and "junk food" because they promote an either/or approach to food. Instead place the focus on achieving a balance.

- Recognize that eating what we label as junk food is seen as normal behavior for adolescents. Girls who eat only "healthy" foods are seen as weird.

- Even though junk food is high in fat, it is also high in nutrients. Take into account that girls are growing and need all the energy they can get.

- Teach the values of strength rather than thinness. Emphasize building strong muscles and bones.

- Look at food as energy. Talk about what happens when your body doesn't have enough fuel.

- Encourage plenty of snacks. Studies show that adolescents get the bulk of their nourishment between meals.

- Find creative ways of compromising around food. Share your feelings about what you like and help her plan what she wants.

- Don't make meals a battleground. Agree to resolve your conflicts in a more neutral place.

- It doesn't matter when you "break the fast." It doesn't have to be first thing in the morning. It could be with a snack at 10:00 A.M.

- Respect when kids are not hungry. They will let you know when they are.

- We place the focus on food. Girls also have to have enough sleep and fluids. Often they are tired because they are dehydrated.

Time Out for Yourself

- **Learn about your own attitudes.** Keep a "feelings" chart for a few days. Each day, write down the positive and negative thoughts that you have had about the food that you eat or the food that you want to eat and don't. This will help you become aware of your underlying beliefs.

- **Learn about food.** Keep a food record for a few days. Write down everything that you eat. Try not to judge yourself in terms of good and bad, only in terms of what you like. What foods do you really want? What foods are missing from your diet? What won't you let yourself have?

 ## Time with Each Other

Be creative. Look through a book on nutrition to see what's missing from your diet, and try something new.

The food you eat:

- What is your favorite food?
- What is your least favorite food?
- Describe a favorite eating experience:
  - Where were you?
  - What did you eat?
  - How did the food taste, smell, feel?
- Describe the perfect meal:
  - Who would be there?
  - Where would it take place?

How food makes you feel:

- Sometimes certain feelings make us want to eat certain things.
    - What kind of food is "angry" food? Why?
    - What kind of food is "sad" food? Why?
- Go through the range of feelings and talk about the associations that you have.

"Good" foods and "bad" foods:

- Make lists of the foods that are considered "good" and "bad."
- What makes them "good" or "bad"?
- How nutritious are they?
- How do you feel when you eat them?

NOTES

1   Marissa Piesman. *Heading Uptown: A Nina Fishman Mystery*. New York: Delacorte Press, 1993, pp. 134-135.
2   Kaz Cooke. *Real Gorgeous. The Truth about Body and Beauty*. NSW, Australia: Allen & Unwin, 1994, p. 25.
3   Gwen Chapman and Heather Maclean. "'Junk Food' and 'Healthy Food': Meanings of Food in Adolescent Women's Culture." *Journal of Nutritional Education*, 1993, No. 25.
4   Health and Welfare Canada. *Nutrition Recommendations: The Report of the Scientific Review Committee*. Canada: Supply and Services, 1990.
5   B.S. Worthington-Roberts and S.R. Williams, eds. *Nutrition through the Life Cycle*. St. Louis: Mosby, 1996, pp. 323-325.

12

Dieting

The Truth about Diets

When I was eleven years old, my mother took me with her to a reducing salon – that was in the good old days before fitness. I looked at the women pedaling furiously on their stationary bicycles, or pushing themselves to touch their toes. I heard them breathing laboriously in the steam room trying to lose their extra pounds. I laughed at the absurdity of their efforts with all of my preadolescence arrogance. The confident child vanished the next year when I began puberty, and was replaced by an insecure adolescent whose precarious sense of self was held hostage by how she looked.

For a large part of my adult life my preoccupation with food and weight took me up and down the scale through a myriad of diets. I became an expert at them all: low-fat, high-fat, grapefruit, thirteen glasses of water – when I failed one weight-loss group I'd move on to the next. I'm not surprised when women tell me that they've had similar experiences. Our lives are regulated by diets and the amount that we weigh. We're either on a diet, in between one, or planning to go on another diet tomorrow. We worry about what we just ate this morning, and plan what we're going to eat tonight. We count calories one day, and fat grams the next. We dream about how different our lives will be when we finally hit that magic number on the scale. While only some of us have struggled with anorexia and bulimia, most of us are caught in the cycle of chronic dieting.

chronic	diet cycle

- We feel fat and tell ourselves that we must do something about it.
- We go on a diet and restrict the amount we eat.
- At some point, we begin to experience the deprivation. We feel angry and rebellious.
- We eat as if our local grocery store were going out of business tomorrow.
- We regain the weight plus some more.
- We feel guilty and bad about ourselves.
- We begin the *diet to end all diets* – all over again.

No matter how much we diet, we can't change our basic body shape. No matter how good we feel when the weight comes off, for 95 percent of us it will probably be back in another two years. Even when we are aware of these statistics we try and try again. Despite our best efforts to lose weight, our dieting makes us fat.

During the last two decades, more and more people have questioned the relationship between dieting and weight. They have shot down our commonly held assumptions that fatness is some kind of abnormality that comes from eating too much. Studies have shown that fat has little to do with willpower and that people who are obese eat the same amount (sometimes even less!) than people who are of normal weight. Fat has more to do with our genetic makeup, and with an internal control system known as the "setpoint," which dictates how much fat a body should carry.[1]

In order to lose weight, we need to eat a lot less than our body needs to function. In a thin person, that is called self-starvation. In the rest of us, it's called dieting. Anorexics take this to an extreme.

Even though it makes us irritable, and interferes with our concentration, and stops us from enjoying what we eat – we do it anyway. It's hard for us to give up dieting. Diets give us structure, an illusion of being in control. Think of the last time you went on a diet. It most likely was at a time when you felt really stressed. We try to control what we eat just when everything else in our life seems to be going haywire. It's scary for us to give ourselves choices. We are afraid that if we allow ourselves to have whatever we want, we'll eat everything in sight.

But our body is smarter than we are. Every time we try to starve our body, our body stays one step ahead of us. It reacts when we give it less fuel than it requires, when we bring our weight down below what it considers normal for who we are. Our body conserves energy by slowing down our metabolism and fights to retain our fat reserves by converting protein from our muscles and our heart. It increases our appetite, so that we eat more and gain weight until our set-point is once again achieved. Because our body tries to protect itself against the next time we try to starve it, it raises our set-point so that we now need fewer calories to maintain our previous weight.[2] It's also difficult for some thin people to gain weight. It takes an adolescent girl approximately 3,200 calories per day to gain 2 pounds in a week.

We all have the hope and the fantasy of the day when finally we will be the ideal body shape. We don't give up dieting without a struggle because giving up dieting means letting go of that dream. We may tell ourselves that our dream is reasonable. After all, we're not trying to look like the models on TV. But before we are ready to give up our diets, we need to understand what being thin means to us. Sometimes we need to grieve for the loss of what might have been before we are ready to get on with what really is.[3]

Girls and Dieting

It is estimated that at any given time, 61 percent of adolescents and young women are dieting.[4] Girls as young as five have been reported to restrict their food intake because they are afraid of getting fat.[5]

"I think that I am too fat," says eleven-year-old Erin. "I eat three times a day like a normal person, but I weigh more than my friends. I've tried to lose weight, but I always put it back. I can't do everything that skinny girls do. Every time I do something I screw up."

Girls are constantly bombarded with dieting messages from the media. They also have to deal with the additional pressure that our own dieting behavior as grown women puts on them to be thin.

"My mother just went on a diet and lost thirty pounds," says thirteen-year-old Christina. "She brags to her friends that we can wear each other's clothes. Now she's after me all the time. She watches what I eat and tells me that if she can eat low-fat, so can I. It's not that I don't want to lose weight, it's that she's trying to control my body."

"On Saturday my mother and I had a big fight," says twelve-year-old Megan. "She made me try on my summer clothes and got mad when they didn't fit. She said that it's because I'm getting fat and she was going to put me on a diet."

Girls entering puberty often deal with the changes in their lives by focusing on the changes in their bodies. When they try to express their discomfort by talking about feeling fat, we try to make them feel better by helping them control their weight.

Says Peggy, the mother of twelve-year-old Megan: "Megan keeps on telling me that she feels fat. I try to tell her to cut out snacking and pay attention to what she eats."

Adds Sarah's mom: "I try to help Sarah by keeping junk food out of the house. Even though she constantly complains that she feels fat, she goes out and eats it with her friends."

We try to pay attention to what girls are eating and even prepare special meals when they feel fat. We try to stop them when they reach for foods that we consider bad. Yet even though girls have asked us to help them, when they reach the point of deprivation or the call of the Oreo cookie sounds, they begin to resent us for not allowing them to have what they want. When girls feel fat and talk about dieting as a way of being in control, we need to help them decode the language of fat and encourage them to talk about what's underneath.

Girls have a tendency to put their trust in what they see as expert opinion. Whatever appears in the media must be true and also good for you just because it is there. We need to provide girls with information about what really happens when we diet and let them know why diets don't work. We also need to talk about how *good* it feels to be well-nourished. This discovery is an incredible one for ex-anorexics and former chronic dieters. We need to offer girls an alternative for the messages they see on TV, and the countless dieting articles in every magazine they read.

It's hard for us to offer girls different choices if we're on diets ourselves and if we think it's really important for us to be thin. It's difficult to allow girls their different body sizes when we see them as reflections of ourselves. Even if we do want to support them, we may not be ready to go off our own diets or give up our "thin" dreams. We then feel guilty because we are stuck in a position where we cannot practice what we preach. Supporting girls doesn't mean changing what's important to us or what's hard for us to do. It does mean being honest about our own relationship to food and weight and looking at the messages that we are passing along. Girls don't expect us to be perfect. They would like us to be real. The bonus in helping girls deal with their weight in a healthy way is that sometimes we end up helping ourselves as well.

what really happens | **when you diet[6]**

Skipping Meals or Decreasing Calories
- Lowers our metabolism so that we store fat more easily from fewer calories.
- Causes us to get the "munchies" for foods that are high in fat and sugar in order to satisfy the brain's and muscles' demand for fuel.
- Lowers our attention span and makes us feel tired and irritable.

Cutting out carbohydrates:
- Takes away our best source of energy and makes us feel tired and moody.
- Gives us the "munchies" so that we take on more fuel.

Cutting out meats without comparable replacement:
- Means that our energy from meals may not last as long.
- Causes us to want fat and sugary foods between meals.
- Puts us at risk of iron deficiency, which makes us feel chronically tired.

Going on diets:
- Diets make you fat. Every time you lose weight by dieting, you gain back more.
- You have a 95 percent probability of regaining the weight within two years.

Fasting:
- Most of the weight that you lose is water that you get back when you begin to eat again.
- Muscle mass decreases – which lowers metabolism.
- Fasting can be very dangerous for some individuals.

Time Out for Yourself

- Chart your life history in terms of weight losses and gains. Draw a line that begins with your birth. Each time you gained weight, draw a peak. Each time you lost weight, draw a valley. Write down your age and what was happening in your life every time you gained and lost.

- Chart your own dieting history. Write down each time you were on a diet and what was going on in your life at that time. Write down the feelings you had.

- Count the number of times that you talk about dieting in one week. This includes not only conversations with others, but things that you tell yourself.

- Throw away your scale – I dare you! If that's too hard to do, put it away for a week. Then put it away for a month.

- Get rid of clothes that don't fit. Most of us have clothes in three sizes: When I Lose Weight, Premenstrual Bloat, and Now.

- Make a list of what you're putting off until you lose weight. Choose one of these things and do it *now*!

 ## Time with Each Other

- Let her know that it's all right for her to be whatever size she is.

- Look at the information about dieting. Talk about fueling our bodies and making us strong.

- Share your own experiences about dieting. Let her know how hard it is for you to stop seeing everything in terms of being thin. Tell her how old you were when you started dieting and what was going on in your life.

- Examine media advertising about diets or weight loss. What do they promise? How do they get us to want to lose weight?

- Pay for your diet talk. Put a quarter in a special jar every time one of you talks about dieting or losing weight. When you have enough money, treat each other to something that doesn't have to do with food.

- Take the tacky diet magnets off your fridge!

NOTES

1 S. Wooley and O. Wooley. "Obesity and Women: A Closer Look at the Facts." *Women's Studies International Quarterly*, 1979, No. 2, pp. 69-79.
2 S. Tenzer. "Fat Acceptance Therapy" in L. Brown and E. Rothblum, eds. *Overcoming Fear of Fat*. New York: Harrington Park, 1989, pp. 39-48.
3 Andria Siegler, "Grieving the Lost Dreams of Thinness," in Catrina Brown and Karin Jasper, eds. *Consuming Passions: Feminist Approaches to Weight Preoccupation and Eating Disorders*. Toronto: Second Story Press, 1993, pp. 151-159.
4 F. Berg. "Who Is Dieting in the United States?" *Obesity and Health*, May/June 1992, pp. 48-49.
5 W. Feldman, E. Feldman and J. Goodman. "Health Concerns and Health Related Behaviour of Adolescents." *Canadian Medical Association Journal*, 1986, No. 134, pp. 489-493.
6 Nutritionist handout, British Columbia Ministry of Health.

13

Our Bodies

One evening many years ago, a friend phoned and asked me if I wanted to go to a movie. It was just before my period, and I was feeling fat and bloated – you know the feeling, when it's hard to do up the zipper and your clothes don't fit. Although all I wanted to do was stay home, she persuaded me to go. A double bill was playing at the theater. The second part was an obscure movie called *The Love Goddesses*.[1] It documented how the definition of female beauty changed from the time that movies were invented until the time that this particular movie was made. Today, I can't remember who phoned me, or the name of the movie we were originally going to see. But I've always remembered how excited I felt when *The Love Goddesses* showed that thin hadn't always been the model for sexuality, and when I saw the big body and lusty energy of Mae West.

Throughout history, the female body, but not the actual female herself, has been the object of worship and adoration. Just go into any museum, or look at any art book, and see the number of paintings and statues that depict the female ideal. While society has always worshipped an ideal body, the ideal hasn't always remained the same.

In the 1890s, the ideal woman was somewhat plump. In the early 20th century, voluptuous was definitely in – as represented in the hourglass figure of the popular, corseted Gibson Girl. Hilde Bruch quotes a French physician who wrote in 1911:

> One must mention here that aesthetic errors of a worldly nature to which all women submit, may want them to stay obese for reasons of fashionable appearance. It is beyond a doubt that in order to have an impressive *décolleté* each woman feels herself duty bound to be fat around the neck, over the clavicle and in her breasts.[2]

During the 1920s, a time of opportunity and freedom for women, the flapper was flat-chested, slim-hipped and androgynous. The emphasis was on her cosmetically decorated face – a mask that prevented her from showing who she really was. Then came the Depression and World War II. As men entered the armed forces, their image of the ideal woman changed. She was now full-bodied and had big shoulders that made her strong enough to take her place in the work force. She also had Betty Grable legs.

In the 1950s, the move to the suburbs was on. Women then tried to emulate Marilyn Monroe. She was someone who was voluptuous and curvaceous. She also had big breasts. In the 1960s and 1970s, the women's movement came into being. But so did Twiggy – a thin, waiflike model who celebrated an anorexic look. Society's obsession with thinness began when she replaced the actress Elizabeth Taylor as the body-type for women to emulate.

These recent fluctuations in the ideal body tell us about women's place in society and about the economics of our time. Women and girls are ranked according to their approximation to the ideal body. Those who are closest to it are revered and given status. When life is precarious and resources are scarce, fat is highly desirable, as it implies wealth and survival. In times of prosperity, with opportunity for women, and social change, body ideals become more restrictive and the ideal woman is childlike, passive and small.[3]

In our society today, thin is promoted as beautiful, healthy, sexual and also as self-disciplined and good. Thin people are perceived to be kind, interesting, outgoing and to have a variety of socially desirable character traits. Just look at how we value movie stars and models, and at how we treat those women who fall outside that image of beauty. The insiders make lots of money. The outsiders are devalued and in turn devalue themselves.

Our Relationship to Our Bodies

We only get one body. It is our area of greatest vulnerability and our greatest source of joy. We express our feelings through our bodies. Try walking around as if you've just won the lottery. Now walk around like you are really depressed. Notice the changes in how you carry yourself. We can make ourselves feel more powerful just by rearranging our shoulders and sitting up straight. The metaphors that we use in our speech also show the emotional range of our bodies. Our face turns white with anger and red with rage. We slump our shoulders with sadness and expand our chests with joy. There are things that we cannot stomach, sometimes we don't have a leg to stand on. We shoulder our responsibilities and hold back our opinions when we're afraid to speak.

Our body is the stage on which we play out many of our experiential dramas. When we feel that we have little or no control over our lives, we try to control our bodies by restricting the food we eat. When we are not able to speak directly about how we feel, our bodies become the context, and the language of fat becomes the means of self-expression. We measure our self-worth and self-value by our physical size and our shape.

We hear a lot about body image, but very little about coming to terms with the body that we have. How we feel about our bodies is ultimately how we really feel about ourselves. How we feel about our bodies is determined in different ways. The most influential messages come from the culture that dictates the kind of external image that we are supposed to project. We also have kinesthetic experiences of our body, which come from how we feel inside.

Finally, there are the things that we learn to tell ourselves about our bodies as we grow up. Coming to terms with our real selves can be a bit of a shock. I remember jumping up and down in yet another fitness class and then comparing myself in the mirror to the women on either side. It suddenly dawned on me that no matter how much I exercised and how little I ate, I would never be transformed into the shape that I desired. My genes would always have the last word in how I looked.

Girls and Their Bodies

Until girls reach puberty they are usually unself-conscious about their bodies. Look at the sensuality of babies squirming with joy at our touch. Watch little girls as they run and jump. See the pleasure that they receive from continuously moving around. It's only when girls reach puberty, and their bodies begin to change, that they lose the inner sense of their bodies and begin to feel shame.

> "Gone are the days when Bonnie used to parade naked around the house," says Jessica. "Now she says 'Don't look at me when I'm dressing.' She's so self-conscious about her body."

Girls are initiated into an anorexic culture during puberty, when they learn that their accumulation of body fat – which is biologically normal and necessary to female development – is judged abnormal by adult society. At a time when they need nourishment the most, they begin to restrict their food intake. Girls in puberty measure themselves against each other and reinforce the message that they must constantly try to change their bodies to fit in.

> "Girls watch each other during lunch time. They say, 'Ooh, are you eating that?!' Even if you don't want to lose weight, people expect you to be trying, or at least to look like you are trying to," says Stacey.

> "It's not fair," laments Jodi. "We don't all start from the same place. We don't have the same build or genes, but we are all expected to look the same!"

> "I watch someone thin walk down the hall," says Mary. "She has an air of confidence because she is thin. You know she feels O.K. about herself."

Girls feel a great deal of ambivalence about their changing bodies as they go through puberty. Boys try to grab their breasts. Adult men and women make comments about their bodies. Girls are taught by TV and magazines that they should look good enough to be noticed. But when that happens, they feel uncomfortable because the attention objectifies their bodies instead of validating their selves.

> "My [seventh grade] teacher was taking orders for T-shirts," says Sarah. "He said to the girls, 'Make sure that you order larger sizes because you all have, you know, [cupping his hands] *bazooms*.'"

> "I remember when I was eleven," says Marcia. "I had a really good friend and her father had gone back to school to get a Ph.D. in counseling. I remember that my body was changing and every time I went over to her house he would ask me if I had hair under my arms yet and if I was getting my period. I remember how weird I felt when he asked me these questions. I soon stopped sleeping over at her house. Even when I became an adult, I would feel uncomfortable whenever I saw him."

When Girls Are Fat

A group of teenage girls were asked on a TV program if they would rather be a rich fat person with a fabulous career or someone who is thin, poor and unemployed. They all looked at the interviewer with horror that she would even suggest there was a choice.[4]

Although girls come in all shapes and sizes, because of our pre-occupation with thinness it's often very difficult for girls who are fat.

> "I have a new pen pal," says Robin. "She keeps writing in her letters about how fat she feels. She asked me to send her my picture and so I did. Then I got hers. She's really skinny. I don't know what she's making such a big deal about. I'm afraid that when she sees my picture she won't want to write to me because I'm fat."

Prejudice against fat is one of our society's remaining socially accepted forms of discrimination. While it may no longer be all right to make comments about someone's race, religion, gender or sexual orientation, it is acceptable to make hurtful comments about their weight. As a result, when girls are fat they're teased and are constantly being criticized and judged.[5]

> "I always wear a T-shirt over my bathing suit when I go to the pool," says Kate. "I don't take it off until I get into the water. Last week I went swimming and I saw these other girls. They were whispering and I knew that it was about me. I don't want to go back to the pool."

Girls suffer from the tyranny of the dressing room.[6] It's hard for them to find clothes when they are big.

> "When I go shopping with my friends nothing ever fits me. The salesladies are all mean to me. None of the clothes that do fit me are the kind of clothes that my friends wear."

As adults, we contribute to the way in which girls come to see themselves. As they go through puberty, we start to see their bodies through a different lens. Where once we looked at girls adoringly in childhood and accepted them the way that they were, we now

become more critical of them as their bodies begin to change.[7]
When girls are fat it is difficult for them to develop self-esteem and
to feel loved and accepted when we and the society around them find
their size – and therefore the girls themselves – unacceptable.[8]
When we try to help girls lose weight in order to fit in, we negate
who they are right now. When we tell girls that it's what's inside that
counts and encourage them to focus on their personalities, we reinforce the myth that you can't be beautiful and fat.

We need to look at our own attitudes toward fat because we
pass them along to girls whether we intend to or not. In one group
that I facilitated, the girls talked about a teacher who brought in
cookies for the students. Realizing that there were not enough to
go around, she said that she would give the cookies to the thin kids
because the fat ones didn't need them!

If it's hard for us to accept ourselves when we are fat or think
that we are fat, we might need help in dealing with our own feelings.
Little girls learn what is valued by how their mothers (and other
mentors) do or do not value themselves.[9] When we have difficulty
accepting our own bodies, it's hard for us to help girls accept theirs.

> "I really worry about Jana," says her mother, Arlene. "She
> reminds me so much of myself when I was her age. I was a
> chubby child and now I'm constantly on a diet. I don't want
> her to go through what I went through. I don't want the
> other girls to tease her. I try to watch what she eats so that
> she won't gain weight."

When Camryn Manheim, star of TV's drama "The Practice,"
dedicated her Emmy to all the fat girls, the audience cheered. For
that moment women in America did not need to suck in their
stomachs to be accepted. We too need to help our fat girls be fat
with dignity. We need to listen to their feelings about being different without trying to fix them. We need to defuse the value
judgments around fat by using the word in the same way that we
would use the words for other characteristics – such as thin, tall,

curly hair, stubborn or creative. We need to let our fat girls know that they are beautiful and that it is all right for them to be who they are. If we are going to start loving our bodies and help girls to continue to love theirs, we need to take the focus away from how we look on the outside and redirect it onto how our bodies feel inside. We need to minimize the emphasis that we place on appearance and start to put our energy into using our bodies and feeling strong.

Using Our Bodies: Exercise and Participation in Sports

We feel better about ourselves when we use our bodies. Exercise makes us stronger and helps us deal with tiredness and stress. It improves our concentration, our posture, our breathing and our digestion. It lowers our cholesterol and blood pressure and helps us build strong bones.[10] When we use our bodies we have an awareness of them that is deeper than the packaging that we see on the outside. When we feel strong in our bodies we feel more in control of our lives. Best of all, when we exercise we are focusing only on ourselves.

> "There's something physiological that makes you feel better," says Helen. "Because I'm a nurse I have a lot of aches and things, and when I go and do my stretching exercises I definitely feel a lot more relaxed and the strain goes away. It's a definite physiological and psychological boost."

Even though it makes us feel good, the only reason that most of us exercise is to lose weight. "We engage in exercise that aims at weight loss as punishment for not looking like the models in the fashion magazines," say Jane Hirschmann and Carol Munter, authors of *When Women Stop Hating Their Bodies*, "and then we rebel against that punishment because we also yearn to be accepted as we are.[11]

As women, we are socialized to not use our bodies. It starts when we are very young. By the time they are six, both sexes believe that boys are better than girls at physical activities. Little girls learn to underestimate their abilities as a result of this belief. This results in their not only having lower fitness and skill levels than boys the same age, but these deficits are compounded with each passing year.[12]

While many girls are physically active in elementary school, their aerobic fitness level (or heart/lung working capacity) starts to decline when they reach adolescence.[13] Physical activity levels also decrease among disabled girls during adolescence after peaking when they are between ten and twelve years old.[14] It's no coincidence that this happens just at the time when girls lose their self-esteem.

As girls go through high school, they pay attention to their bodies by trying to make themselves look good. The older they get, the less importance physical activity has in their lives. A recent survey found that while only 30.6 percent of high school freshman girls participate in sports, that number drops even lower – to 17.3 percent – by their senior year.[15] It seems that girls have their periods every time they have PE!

Girls stop using their bodies for many reasons. High school gym or PE does not address the realities of their lives or their changing bodies. Often there is not enough time for girls to shower and change so that girls who want to be physically active must go around sweaty for the rest of the day. Even if showers are available, the pressure to be thin makes girls self-conscious about their bodies and thus reluctant to undress in front of each other. Girls who have never had breasts before now have to run around the gym without the support of an athletic bra because they are unaware of its existence. Many girls give up when classes do not honor different body types and plan for them accordingly.

Girls see sports differently than boys. Boys tend to see sports in terms of achievement, so they are more likely to learn from their mistakes. And because rules and competition are part of male development, participation in sports is viewed as a valuable part of their lives. While many girls succeed at competition, the emphasis on connection always comes first. Girls whose skill levels are low tend not to participate because the traditional militaristic form of sports instruction is not part of their culture.

Even girls who want to participate in more physical activity often find it difficult because they have to take a back seat here to the boys. In elementary school, they are relegated to the sidelines in the schoolyard while boys get the lion's share of the playing space. In high school, boys get first shot at the playing fields and ice rinks that traditionally have been considered their domain.

> "There are a number of girls in our community who want to play hockey," says Lara's mother. "Whenever we insist on having ice time for them we are accused of taking the ice time away from the boys. It always seems that fairness is a one-way street and that we are going in the wrong direction."

When girls try to join in, they are intimidated. Sometimes they are harassed.

> "I want to try out for the basketball team," says eleven-year-old Ariel, "but I'm not that good. The boys won't let me play with them at recess because I'm not as good as they are. Even when they let me play they push and shove me and won't throw the ball."

It is important for girls to use their bodies when they are young and to continue to be physically active as they go through adolescence. Just thirty minutes of physical activity a day can increase peak bone mass in early adulthood and delay the onset of osteoporosis[16] and reduce the risk of coronary heart disease, diabetes[17] and breast cancer[18] in adulthood. Girls who are physically active are found to be healthier, less susceptible to stress and to depression, are more independent, and have greater self-esteem.[19] They are more at ease and accepting of their bodies. They are more likely to delay their first experience of intercourse and, later on, more likely to practice safe sex.[20] They are also less likely to smoke.[21]

In order for girls to remain physically active, programs must be designed for their specific body type, and set at a skill level that offers them a measure of success. If girls are given a safe environment where they trust that it is okay to make a mistake and they know that the team is there to support them, they will participate in and benefit from team sports.[22]

Girls need to be taught that physical activity is not just about track or baseball. They need to be introduced to other forms of activity and movement such as dance, skating, gymnastics, yoga and martial arts. These activities are often overlooked or discounted. Female dancers, gymnasts and skaters often have a schizophrenic experience. They are athletes who participate in very physically demanding sports. On the other hand, their athletic abilities and strength can be overlooked and negated as the emphasis focuses on their femininity and cuteness.

Girls need more role models to look up to. Right now fewer than 5 percent of newspapers' sports pages are devoted to women. Female athletes receive less than 10 percent of the coverage on TV.[23] In *TV Guide's* list of "TV's Greatest Sports Moments," only three and a half featured women: Torvill and Dean's Gold medal-winning performance at the 1984 Winter Olympics (#10); Kerri Strug's courageous vault at the 1996 Atlanta games (#14); Bonnie Blair's history-making performance at the 1994 Olympics when she became the first American woman to win four gold medals (#20); and Joan Benoit's victory in the first Olympic marathon for women in 1984 (#26).[24]

Yet while change is slow, it is happening. A record number of women competed in the 1996 Olympic games – 1,000. Forty-two percent of the U.S. team were women, while women on the Canadian team outnumbered the men. When women compete in the same number of team sports as men in Sydney in 2002, they will challenge the assumption that sport and physical activity in general belongs to boys and men.

Girls need to see more women participating as athletes, as coaches, and on teams. Inclusion of softball in the Atlanta Olympics, and the focus on women's basketball, volleyball and rowing, displayed a range of body types and activities, and emphasized strength and skill. This allowed girls to see that women can be strong and competitive, and still be connected to each other. The American women at Atlanta – the first generation to grow up under Title IX – demonstrated by their success the benefits of equal access to resources and training.

When girls are young we need to instill in them a lifelong commitment to use their bodies. If girls do not participate in sports by the time they are ten, there is only a 10 percent chance that they will participate when they are twenty-five.[25] That doesn't mean they have to become world-class athletes – but that they learn that physical activity is fun and something that everybody can do successfully. We can help by encouraging them to participate and by becoming role models for them by being active ourselves.

> "I don't think exercise should be something that you don't like doing," says Jessica. "I vary it at times. I like to get out and walk. I go to the gym or, you know, a whole lot of different things. If you make it a real punishment routine it's not fun anymore. It has to be a treat, too. You're treating yourself and it feels doubly nice that way.

 ## Time Out for Yourself

- **Get to know your body.** Which parts of your body do you feel belong to you? Which parts of your body don't? Where do you feel strong? Where do you feel most vulnerable? Which parts of your body hold your anger, your tension? Which parts of your body do you have the most difficulty with? Which parts of your body are painful? Which parts give you joy? (This exercise might be difficult. We are not used to thinking about our bodies in such terms. Have a little patience and curiosity. The answers won't come all at once.)

- **Look at your own relationship to exercise.** Some of us treat exercise like diets. We start with good intentions, and we're gung-ho until we poop out. We stop doing it and feel guilty. Then it takes a long time for us to start again. Others of us get pretty obsessive about exercise. We do it after every time we eat. If this description fits you, then you need to take a look at your relationship with your own body and your attitudes toward your own weight.

- **Start using your body.** You don't need to join a team or become an Olympic athlete. Going for a walk also makes you feel good about yourself.

- **Look at what's holding you back.** What are some of the things that you would enjoy? What's holding you back? Sometimes we don't do things because we feel that we are too fat or that we will fail.

 ## Time with Each Other

- **Cover your mirrors for a week.** Consider what life would be like if you didn't always determine what you were feeling by checking out how you looked.

- **Fight the body police.** Often people feel that they have the right to make comments about our bodies – especially if we are fat, or just developing. Role-play some of these situations, and practice what you can say.

- **Dig out the photos and look at your genes.** Who do you look like? Whose hips do you have, whose height? What family traits do each of you exhibit?

- **Compare yourself to birds and flowers.** All of us come in different shapes and sizes, just like flowers and birds. If you were a flower, what kind would you be? Why?

  What other kinds of flowers are there in your family? Try the same thing with birds.

- **Discover your body type.** While bodies are all individual, they can be loosely broken down into three body types:

  - Endomorphs tend to have rounder body types, with more body fat and softer curves.

  - Ectomorphs are slim, less curvy and more angular.

  - Mesomorphs are muscular, with wide shoulders and slim hips.

- **Explore different physical activities.** What kinds make you feel good? What kinds make you feel awkward?

- **Use your bodies.** Go for walks together. This is a good time to talk. Turn on a tape or CD or the radio and sing really loud. Singing is a great emotional release. Put on loud music and dance, dance, dance.

Notes

1   *The Love Goddesses*. 83 minutes. Saul J. Turell, director, 1965.

2   Hilde Bruch. *Eating Disorders: Obesity, Anorexia Nervosa and the Person Within*. New York: Basic Books, 1973, p. 18.

3   Beth MacInnis. "Fat Oppression" in Catrina Brown and Karin Jasper, eds. *Consuming Passions: Feminist Approaches to Weight Preoccupation and Eating Disorders*. Toronto: Second Story Press, 1993, pp. 69-79.

4   WTN: "You, Me and the Kids." Episode on body image.

5   Susan Kano. *Making Peace with Food: Freeing Yourself from the Diet/Weight Obsession*. New York: Harper & Row, 1989.

6   Jane R. Hirschmann and Carol H. Munter. *When Women Stop Hating Their Bodies: Freeing Yourself from Food and Weight Obsession*. New York: Fawcett Columbine/Ballantine Books, 1995, pp. 12, 86.

7   Teresa Pitman and Miriam Kaufman, M.D. *The Overweight Child: Promoting Fitness and Self-Esteem*. Toronto: Firefly Books, 2000.

8   Hirschmann and Munter.

9   *American Journal of Health Promotion*, 1996, Vol. 10, pp. 171-174.

10 Ibid.

11 Hirschmann and Munter.

12 Wendy Dahlgren. *A Report of the National Task Force on Young Females and Physical Activity*. Ottawa, Canada: Department of Fitness and Amateur Sport, 1988.

13 Kaz Cooke. *Real Gorgeous. The Truth about Body and Beauty*. NSW, Australia: Allen & Unwin, 1994, pp. 72-74, 216.

14   *Pediatric Exercise Science*, 1994, vol. 6, pp. 168-177.

15   U.S. Department of Health. Youth Risk Behavior Survey, 1990.

16   *Medicine and Science in Sports and Exercise*, 1996, Vol. 28, pp. 105-113.

17   U.S. Department of Health and Human Services. *Report of the Surgeon General: Physical Activity and Health*, 1996.

18   *Journal of the National Cancer Institute*, 1994.

19   Colton and Gore. "Risk Resiliency and Resistance: Current Research on Adolescent Girls," Ms. Foundation, 1991.

20   *The Women's Sports Foundation Report: Sport and Teen Pregnancy*, May 1998.

21   *Medicine and Science in Sports and Exercise*, 1996, Vol. 27 pp. 1639-1645.

22   *On the Move: Increasing Participation of Girls and Women in Physical Activity and Sports*. Vancouver, BC: Premier's Sports Awards Program, 1993.

23   Cooke.

24   *TV Guide*, July 8-11, 1998.

25   Linda Bunker, University of Virginia, 1989.

14

Friends

There is absolutely, positively, nothing in the world as great as a best friend. Even when we have husbands, lovers, or boyfriends, nobody takes the place of the special women in our lives. A friend who likes you helps you like yourself. She is someone who listens to your problems with the right amount of empathy, and shares hers in return. She is someone you run to phone to share the latest news – even if you saw her just the day before. If your good friends live elsewhere, and you don't see them very often in person, there is still something about the quality of women's friendships that makes it easy for us to pick up where we left off.

Sometimes we have one or two very special friends who remain our friends throughout our lives. They are people with whom we share our history. They provide us with perspective and continuity. They are able to remind us that the things we worry about now are the same things we worried about before. We also make new friends throughout our lives. We go through different life stages and experiences, and as our interests change, so do the people in our lives. Sometimes we move away and have to start all over again. Sometimes our friendships end because of disagreements or hurts that we don't have the skills to fix.

Because we know the value of our friendships, we worry when our girls don't fit in – when we feel that they don't have enough friends.

> "I worry about Carol," says Rena. "She's such an individual and doesn't really have a best friend. The school that she goes to is small and her interests are different from the other kids. I had a lot of friends when I was growing up and my friends are important to me now. I want the same thing for her."

Although we want the best for our girls, we have to be careful in how we try to help them. When we encourage girls to join organized activities, they often see this as pressure – not as something that they would really like to do. It helps if we go with them when girls are younger. As they get older we need to let them know that it's okay to try things and not go back again if they don't like it. Girls feel pressured if they think that they can't take the time to feel things out, and unheard or misunderstood if they think they can't just say no.

One of the biggest beefs girls have is that their parents assume they can play with or relate to girls they have never met before – just because they are the same age. Girls need time to check each other out and to negotiate the complicated rules of friendship. While the desire to make friends may be very strong, the fear of being seen as uncool is often much stronger.

> "Last summer we spent three weeks at the lake," says Colleen. "The first week there were no other girls Liane's age and she was very lonely. The second week a family arrived with a thirteen-year-old daughter. I kept telling Liane to go and talk to her but she didn't want to make the first move. Finally one day they ended up going swimming at the same time. After that they were inseparable until we went home."

Girls' second biggest beef is when their teachers pose as social workers and try to get them to reach out to someone just because she is shy, or needs a friend, or is going through a hard time. When girls are told to act with compassion, they end up resenting the outsider even more. We need to remember how emotionally charged the issue of friendship is for girls. It's hard for them to include someone else on demand, when they are constantly worried about how they themselves fit in.

Making and Keeping Friends

Sometimes girls find themselves in a position where their best friend moves away, or changes in their family mean that they have to move to a new community and go to a different school. Girls entering high school often find that their former friends have changed. For many girls this is a very lonely time. It's hard for some girls to make new friends. Even when they do, their friendships don't proceed as smoothly as they would like them to.

> "My best friend moved to Boston," says Rachel as she fights back tears, "and my second best friend moved to Chicago. I don't have anyone to talk to. I talk to my mom but it's not the same. She's a mom."

> "I used to be good friends with Sarah," says Lara. "Then she got angry because I didn't do things her way. Now Melissa won't talk to me. She found someone else. I'm so scared of doing something wrong that I don't say anything anymore."

Often girls distance themselves from one another because they don't have the skills to deal with conflicts or with hurt feelings when they occur. When girls are unsure why their friendships have ended, they often assume that it must be something they have said or done.

"If your friend is mad at you and you said you're sorry and she doesn't forgive you," asked Carolyn, "do you think she hates you because you gained weight?"

As girls reach adolescence, their friendships are likely to be closer and more intense than at any other time in their lives. At this stage of their development, girls have the cognitive and emotional skills to understand another person's point of view and can understand how the other person thinks and feels.[1] While these skills help girls develop intimacy between them, by allowing them to share their deepest feelings and thoughts, they also have a down side. Like first-year psychology students, girls overanalyze the other person's behavior, feelings and motives. They overempathize with the other person often at their own expense. Because they are socialized to be kind and nice, they withhold their own feelings for fear of hurting the other person and, in the process, run the risk of losing themselves. When girls focus solely on the other person, they lose sight of their own qualities and try to reinvent themselves to fit their image of the ideal friend.

In the grade eight groups that I've been involved with, most of the girls' issues centered around interpersonal dynamics. We taught the girls communication skills and encouraged them to express how they felt. We had the girls make lists of what they wanted in a friend and compare this to a list of how they thought they should be:

What I Want in a Friend	How I Should Be
• Same views as you	• Help people
• Listens to you	• Skinny
• Someone I can talk to	• Sense of humor
• Be there for you	• Able to talk about things
• Doesn't have too many problems	• More fun
• Patience	• Less picky
• Not popular and so has time	• Easygoing
• Care about me more than about them	• Confident, less touchy
• Dependable and reliable	• More talkative

The girls learned that no matter how hard they try to please or satisfy the other person, they can't control what she will ultimately do. Friendships are not just between two people. We bring along our entire histories with our parents and siblings and our experiences in the world into every interaction that we have. Despite our best intentions, the other person's buttons sometimes get pushed. And because she doesn't have the awareness or the insight or the skills to deal with our baggage, she finds a reason for moving away.

Helping and Overhelping Friends

Helping or taking care of others is a wonderful part of who girls are. But sometimes they become so engrossed in the other person's feelings and experiences that they begin to neglect their own. They become so concerned with the other person that they forget about their own feelings and needs. They step outside their own boundaries and break the other person's fences down.

When girls step outside their own boundaries, they begin to feel powerless, resentful and angry – or all three. This happens when they want to help someone but helping them creates a conflict between their own needs and their friend's. Sometimes their friend's problem may be too big or too much for girls to handle, but they don't know that or they feel guilty saying so. Sometimes they are scared that they won't do the right thing, or become resentful because they feel their friend is asking for too much. They try to deal with their discomfort by telling their friend what to do, in the hope that the problem will go away. When their friend doesn't follow this advice, girls feel angry and pressured and misunderstood.

Girls need help with boundaries. They want to be there for their friends, but if they are overhelping them, and feeling trapped or panicky, they need us to help set the limits for them. In one group thirteen-year-old Cara talked about her struggle with balancing her own needs and still trying to help her friend Beckie whose parents were getting a divorce. After Beckie began to spend more and more time at Cara's, she told Cara that she wanted to move in.

"Beckie's my best friend," said Cara. "I really wanted to be there for her, but I didn't want her to live with us. She was so angry and upset all the time and I was afraid that if I said no to her that I was going to hurt her and make her feel worse."

Cara's mother came to the rescue. She helped Cara by saying to her, "Tell Beckie your mother won't let you." "My mother won't let me" absolves girls of their responsibility and allows them to get out of situations they otherwise can't handle.

Sometimes girls want to help their friends but the problem is too big for them. Such a case happened when Jodi and her friends saw Alison throwing up in the bathroom. When Alison swore them to silence, they were caught in a dilemma. On the one hand, they wanted to be there for Alison. On the other, they worried about her health. When Jodi finally told her mother, her mother took the problem out of Jodi's hands by speaking to Alison's mother.

The Importance of Peer Groups

As girls become adolescents, the bonds they establish with each other help them fill the need for intimacy that develops as their relationship with their parents begins to change and they become more autonomous. Girls sit together during lunch, they hang out together after school and do things together on the weekends. They share and examine every detail of their lives. Even when girls are not physically together they remain joined via the telephone cord.

The peer group is very important to girls and has a lot of influence on them. Girls measure themselves against the way others see them. They use this feedback to form opinions about their abilities and skills. The peer group gives them an opportunity to test their opinions, feelings and attitudes against those of other girls and to decide which of their parental values they will accept or reject. The peer group also provides girls with emotional security – they see their friends sharing the same problems and having the same way of looking at the world.

No one peer group is suitable for all girls. Girls choose the group whose members are most like them. Then the group tries to make everybody be the same. Girls expect each other to follow set rules of friendship and to act, talk and dress in a certain way. Those girls who don't fit in, or are different, are often made fun of and rejected by their peers.

As adults we worry about the influence of the peer group. We imagine other girls telling our girls what to do. The girls themselves, however, don't see it quite that way. In fact they are quite offended that we think they can be influenced by someone else. Girls evaluate each other in terms of equality, which they see as sameness. They feel that they alone make the choice to adapt their behavior so that they can be equal to their friends. Eleven-year-old Kate explained this best when we were talking about smoking.

> "I know that smoking is bad for you," she said. "It smells, and your lungs get black. Right now, I don't think that I would ever smoke. But that may change in high school. If all of my friends smoked, I would have to – if I wanted to be equal. If they didn't, then neither would I. It's like R-rated movies – my mother doesn't understand why I need to watch them, because they are so bad. It's not that I want to see them, it's that if I don't, I'm not being equal to my friends. I couldn't talk about the things that they talked about and then I would feel left out."

When we talk to our girls about peer pressure we need to do so in terms of what it means to their culture instead of what it means to us. We can begin by acknowledging the importance of being equal, and explore with them other people that they can be equal to and other ways of being equal that make them feel good about themselves instead of engaging in behaviors that put them at risk.

The Dark Side of Friendship

Do you remember how it was in elementary school? Inseparable from our best friend, we promised each other that we would be friends forever. And then our best friend went and found someone new. We found another best friend, and most likely at some point did the same thing to her.

As girls approach adolescence they are taught that dealing with conflict will kill off their relationships – that the other person will reject them if they are not continuously caring and nice. But it's impossible to have a relationship with someone else without ever feeling hurt and anger, and these feelings don't just disappear. One way that girls deal with these feelings is by redirecting them against themselves and encoding them in the language of fat. Girls also express their feelings indirectly. When they cannot be honest with one another, their friendships develop a dark side. Around the time that they are eleven or twelve, hurtful secrets emerge. Girls speak about their friends behind each other's backs. They write notes about them in school. They tell stories that get passed around to everyone – except the girl who is being talked about.

> "Some of the girls in my class keep notebooks and they write things in them about everyone else," says thirteen-year-old Stephanie. "Then at lunch time, they all sit together and pass around their notebooks and laugh."

While girls are capable of achieving the closest intimacy, they can also practice the most exquisite cruelty. Given the importance to girls of connection, it's not surprising that their choices of weapons are ridicule and exclusion.

> "This year, I have had a lot of problems with friends," says twelve-year-old Anna. "Some of my friends I don't like that much and some of my friends are nice but also mean. Right now I'm confused, because I don't know if my so-called friends like me. They have been writing notes without me and doing out-of-school activities without me, too."

When girls talk about the reasons why they exclude each other, they list being immature, wearing the wrong clothes, and being different.

> "The girls in my class don't want to play with me during recess," says eleven-year-old Jodi. "They tease me because I am really good at track and field."

Sometimes girls are excluded because they have broken the rules of friendship. In one grade seven class, the teacher was concerned because she thought that the girls were having difficulty with the fact that one of the students was anorexic and kept alternating between going into the hospital and returning to the class. When the school nurse and I divided the girls into smaller discussion groups, we both found that the discomfort was not around the anorexia but because this one particular girl had broken the friendship rules. She was too direct with the boys and not concerned enough with the girls.

> "She calls us and tells us that she wants to know what everybody is doing, but she never asks us how we feel."

> "She calls the boys and tells them that she likes them and asks them who they like in the class."

In each grade there are girls who are designated as the popular girls. Sometimes popular girls are more physically developed and seem to be more sexually aware and more cool. Sometimes they have other attributes that the rest of the girls want – they are the smartest or the most athletic.

> "Carla was my best friend for a while," says eleven-year-old Erin. "She was very nice. Then she was with Lindsay. They pretend that they are really higher than everyone else and they're the coolest. And they have their little enclosed area

and they tell people 'We don't want you back there' and this one girl, they make faces at her all the time. They raise their eyebrows and they scrunch up their noses. They're very mean to her."

While popular girls get their power by forming cliques and by excluding the other girls, it's important to remember that popular girls experience and are reacting to the same insecurities as the girls who are trying to emulate them.

"I try to tell Nikki about my own experiences whenever she worries about not being popular," said Cathy. "I was a popular girl, but I always felt and sometimes still feel fat, ugly and not good enough for any relationships. Being popular didn't make me value myself more, although everyone assumes that it should."

In the game of exclusion there is always a different victim. Because the rest of the girls will do anything not to be excluded, they will readily betray their friends – and subsequently end up feeling betrayed. In one grade six group, the dynamics around inclusion and exclusion were so intense that it was almost impossible to break them and refocus the girls. The co-facilitator and I watched as each week one of the girls complained that she was being picked on and at how eagerly she rejoined her tormentors the next week to pick on somebody else.

It is very difficult for us to deal with the dark side of girls' friendships. Telling girls to stop telling secrets or excluding one another just means that the behaviors go underground. We can't force girls to be friends with one another. We can, however, give them different weapons to use when their friendships become derailed. We can validate their feelings when girls are being excluded by their friends and provide them with a more realistic perspective when it seems to them that it will never end. We can defuse the power of exclusion by naming it and discussing it in the classroom.

This doesn't mean telling girls that what they are doing is bad. It means giving them a context for their behavior and offering them different ways of dealing with their disputes. One of the most effective ways of dealing with secrets and exclusion is to teach girls (and boys) conflict resolution skills when they are young, and to regularly set aside time in the classroom so that they can practice these skills and incorporate them into their lives. Teaching girls good communication skills also means helping them to recognize their feelings and encouraging them to express them. When girls can deal with each other directly, their sense of fairness and empathy often proves stronger than their need to inflict pain.

Sometimes, despite all our efforts, cliques get carried to an extreme, as when groups of girls begin to gang up on one another. In one school, a group of seventh grade girls were phoning other girls in the class and threatening them. It got so bad that the police had to be called in. In some cases, girls are turning their anger outward and are dealing with their feelings by beating up other girls.

While we don't want to interfere in girls' conflicts, we have to be aware that girls need our protection. One father that I talked to said that at his daughter's school the cliques were so strong that she was constantly being victimized. He was finally forced to take her out of the school. Schools have to keep girls safe. If they can't, then girls need us to step in – even if they protest when we do so.

Relationships with Boys

In my work with women, I often ask them how they came to be in a relationship with the person that they are with. Nine times out of ten the answer is, "He was interested in me." As adult women, we put more effort into researching a used car than we do into choosing a mate. We're so busy pleasing the man in our lives so he won't reject us that we forget to ask ourselves if he is really someone we want to be with in the first place. In exchanging "me" for "we," we never actually look at who "he" is – at those qualities in him that we are drawn to, as well as those that make us want to pull away.

As girls enter the world of heterosexual relationships, their behavior is very much like our own. As soon as they become interested in boys they ask, "Does he like me?" instead of, "Do I like him?" They become the choosee rather than the chooser. They also think that if someone likes them they are not allowed to say no. When I work with girls, I try to redirect their focus away from worrying about being wanted to thinking about what they want. Encouraging them to talk about the qualities of a particular boy helps them decide whether they are interested in this boy as a person, instead of idealizing him as a boyfriend and losing themselves.

Girls focus on boys to the exclusion of their own sense of reality and sometimes their own personal safety. Because girls and boys occupy different cultures, they view the same encounter from totally different perspectives. Chapter 10 on sexuality talks about how boys have sex with girls who are having love. Yet when something goes wrong, or when boys begin to distance themselves or reject them outright, girls attribute the loss of connection they are experiencing to something specific that they themselves have done wrong. Instead of looking at how they can change the relationship, they try to change themselves. They are convinced that if only they were prettier, skinnier, blonder, etc., the relationship would be a success.

> "Why is it," asks fifteen-year-old Emily, "that when you like a guy and you finally get him, you feel you're not good enough for him? Then you start to do things that make you look better. And then you realize that you don't look better, and you worry all the time."

When twelve-year-old Michelle wrote a story about rejection, she quite accurately depicted what most of us do with men:

> Maggie enjoyed the dance and she felt close and warm. "I love you, Brian," she thought, wishing to yell it out. Then, "Brian thinks I'm fat and ugly and he just asked me to dance to be nice," Maggie thought as the song ended.

A week later Maggie found out that a beautiful girl had asked Brian out and he had said no. "He really meant it," Maggie thought. "Maybe I'm not so fat and ugly after all."

The best way that we can help girls is to take the focus off the boy and bring it back to themselves.

---

consider these questions | *early* **in a relationship***

How do I know if someone loves me?

Is this person I care about someone who:
- listens to me?
- considers my feelings and ideas?
- shares my interests, activities and beliefs?
- enjoys spending time with me?
- remembers little things that are important to me?
- lets me be first sometimes?
- values and takes care of himself?
- does everything he can to help me reach my full potential?

How do I know if someone could hurt me?

Is this person I care about someone who:
- ignores my feelings and wishes?
- teases and ridicules me about things that are important to me?
- doesn't keep my confidences?
- ignores me or pretends not to hear me?
- acts more friendly when we are alone than when his friends are around?
- sulks when I don't do what he wants?
- often shows anger and uses threats or violence in the relationship to get his own way?
- encourages or pressures me to do things that make me uncomfortable?

*Excerpted from the pamphlet, *Dating Violence Prevention* (Canadian Red Cross).

We need to help girls decode the language of fat and express the feelings that lie underneath. Often these are feelings of disappointment, insecurity and anger. We also need to take the focus off romance and help girls make the other person real. We can talk about who the boy is, and help them articulate what they want from a relationship.

Some girls get into relationships with boys who are abusive. There are many reasons why they don't leave. Girls who come from families where there is violence often believe that this is the way boys are supposed to be, and they have no choice if they want a boyfriend. Some girls are afraid to hurt the boy's feelings. Not being liked is more terrifying than being hurt. Some girls believe that if the boy is abusive, it must be their fault.

Because their primary concern is so often pleasing boyfriends, many girls have difficulty saying no when they don't want to have sex. Even if they know about safe sex, they will risk pregnancy and sexually transmitted diseases rather than displease their boyfriend by insisting that he wear a condom.

We can teach girls what makes relationships abusive, so that they know what to look out for when they begin to date. We can also teach girls how to say "no." We can support them when they try to assert themselves so that they can begin to make healthy choices for themselves.

Strategies to Consider

- Help girls resolve conflict. As long as girls are not in danger, it's best when we don't intervene. However, you can begin by validating her feelings and then helping her sort them out. This means helping her move from "Mary is such a bitch," or "Andrew is such a nerd," to "I felt angry when Mary/Andrew ..." [It might be helpful to review chapter 8 on communication skills.]

- Attack the behavior, not the friend. Help her describe the behavior that is hurtful to her. Girls fight and make up with great frequency. The girl or boyfriend you criticize today may be her best friend tomorrow.

- Try not to overanalyze. It helps to have a context for the other person's behaviors. But we have to be careful that we don't spend all of our time analyzing and understanding them and in the process negate or deny our own feelings.

- Role-play the conflict. Girls love to act things out. Ask her to coach you so that you can take the part of the girl or boy with whom she is having the conflict. How would the other girl or the boy act? What would she or he say? Role-playing allows us to say what we need to say without worrying about the other person's feelings. It allows us to try out different endings and to practice different solutions.

- Provide a perspective. When girls have conflicts with their friends it sometimes feels to them as if it will never end. We can provide them with a more realistic perspective.

- Share yourself. You know what to do here!

 ## Time with Each Other

Be curious about your friendships. Friendship is like a dance. Some things make you move closer. Some things make you move away. It's always interesting for us to know why we are friends with certain people and what things about them make us want to move away. You can do this exercise together and talk about her friends. Or you can do it separately. It might be interesting for you to apply it to some of your own relationships:

Girlfriends

- What's the best part of having a best friend?
- What is the hardest part?
- What are the similarities between you?

- What are the differences?
- What interests do you share?
- What are the things that you disagree about?
- What are the three qualities that draw you to her?
- What are the three qualities that make you move away?
- What do you suppose are the qualities in you that drew her to you?
- What do you think bugs her about you?
- What are some of the problems that you have with your friend?
- How do you resolve them?

Boyfriends

- What kind of person is the boy you are presently interested in?
- How are you alike, and how are you different?
- Describe your ideal boyfriend – his appearance, personality, likes or dislikes?
- How would this ideal boyfriend make you feel?
- How would you interact with one another?
- What kinds of things would you do together?
- How would you want him to treat you?
- How would you want him to be with your friends?

NOTE

1   Diane F. Paplia and Sally Wendkos Olds. *A Child's World: Infancy through Adolescence*. New York: McGraw Hill. 1990, pp. 578-579.

15

The Lessons of the Classroom

The very first day of grade one is the same all over. The morning bell rings. Girls hold hands and giggle. Boys jostle one another as they line up. For many girls, this routine will be familiar. They have already learned how to sit quietly, work cooperatively and please others. They know that they can look forward to basking in praise in return for helping the teacher. During the early school years, girls do better than boys because they have the right tools for the job. They have much better social skills and are better at communication. The structure of their female brain gives them a greater disposition to developing the kinds of auditory and motor skills important in learning to read.[1]

Starting school can be a very different experience for boys. Raised to be active, aggressive and independent, it's difficult for them to sit still for long periods of time or to raise their hands whenever they want to speak. They don't know how to contain their energy or to work in groups without poking and jostling one another. During the early years of elementary school, the same visual and spatial skills that will give boys the edge later on are not very helpful when it comes to learning to read. Boys account for four out of every five children with reading disorders such as dyslexia. Ninety-five percent of children diagnosed as hyperactive are boys.[2] Many of them tend to act out their frustrations in class. Like the girls, boys also want the teacher's praise. Unlike the girls, who try to please, boys attempt to get the teacher's attention through competition. He who is the loudest will have the best chance of being heard!

The teacher faces this brand new day with a certain measure of excitement, anticipation and apprehension. With anywhere from fifteen to thirty children in the class (depending on the school system), she is expected to teach the basics. She also has to make sure that the kids are not bouncing off the classroom walls. She is grateful for the cooperation of the girls. They are so much easier to handle. The boys, on the other hand, need her more. They are also more likely to get out of control. The teacher gives the boys more resources and attention, and consistently goes the extra mile for them. She tries to tell herself that because the girls are quieter, they really don't need her as much. Girls pay a price for peace in the classroom – because the teacher's extra efforts with the boys usually come at their expense. While the teacher may like the girls better, she ends up directing her best teaching efforts toward the boys.[3]

The teacher asks a question. The hands shoot into the air. The girls hold theirs up politely until overlooked, then lower them in defeat. The boys, on the other hand, wave their arms. They lift their bodies out of their seats. "Ooh, ooh," they moan – their behavior urging the teacher to "pick me, pick me, pay attention to me!" If that doesn't work, their voices get stronger, and then in frustration they begin to call out loud.

The Lessons of Inequality

According to Myra and David Sadker, authors of *Failing at Fairness: How Our Schools Cheat Girls*, boys receive most of the attention in the classroom.[4] Boys call out eight times more often than girls. Teachers accept this kind of behavior – and respond to the urgency that seems to be underneath it – even when what the boys have to say is irrelevant to the discussion. When girls call out, they are reminded of the rules and told to raise their hands.[5] After a while, the girls give up in frustration. The typical girl "crosses her legs, folds her arms across her chest and hunches forward toward her desk, seemingly to shrink into herself … Meanwhile, the boys sprawl in their chairs, stretching their legs long, expanding into the available space."[6]

When teachers call on the boys, they prompt them, and give them hints to help them find the right answer if their original response was incorrect. When they interact with boys, they praise them and correct them. They help them and criticize them. They encourage them and give them specific feedback. "You can do it Jimmy, just try a little harder." "See, you might have missed four questions, but you got six right." "Your answer here was wrong, but that's probably because you were tired. Now just try it again." "Your essay was interesting, Bobby. It had a lot of action. The subject was quite real. You just need work on spelling." All of these activities help boys acquire the necessary skills for learning.

Girls receive less time, less help and fewer challenges from their teachers. They are called upon less often in class and are passed over if they don't answer right away. This means that they lose their chance to engage with her in the learning process. When teachers praise girls, it is usually with empty words that give them little information about what they did right, what they did wrong, and what they need to do to correct it.[7] "Your work is so neat, Peggy." "That's good, dear." "You look so pretty, Janice." "What a nice dress." Without specific feedback and the opportunity to practice, girls never get to recognize and name their abilities or develop confidence in themselves. They don't have a chance to learn the strategies from which to learn or correct their mistakes, and they come to believe that when they do something wrong, it is because there is something wrong with them.[8]

Speaking out in class is important. It acknowledges that the student is important and has a right to speak and to be heard. The more you talk in class, the more opportunities you have to be praised, to know your strengths and abilities, and to learn to experience being wrong as an educational tool instead of a personal deficiency.[9] Each time that the teacher addresses a boy instead of a girl, and each time she treats them differently, the lesson that she teaches is that girls are worth less and that their opinions are not as important as those of the boys. Eventually the girls give up and come to believe their negative voice, the one that tells them they are stupid – and if they fail it's all their own fault.

The lessons of inequality become ingrained in the classroom. Even when teachers do make an attempt to correct the imbalance, they are told by the girls that they are not being fair to the boys![10] Yet equal opportunity is not a contest or a trade-off. It means treating everybody with respect and ensuring that everyone has a say and a place.

When Boys Have Ability and Girls Have Luck

As girls go through school they lose confidence in their ability to do math. Even when girls start out doing as well as boys, those who begin to see math as a male subject begin to do less well compared to the boys. According to a study done by the American Association of University Women (AAUW), about one-third of elementary school girls and one-half of the boys say that they are good in math. By high school, one out of four boys and one out of seven girls still believe that they can do well.[11] Because girls are not taught how to learn from their mistakes, the first time they experience a failure in math they subsequently begin to achieve at a much lower level. They see their failure as a sign that they are stupid and can't do the work. When girls do well they, and their teachers, see their success as the result of luck, or because they have tried really hard. When boys fail, it is seen as a result of bad luck or laziness. When they do well it is attributed to their ability.[12]

Doing well in math and science can mean the difference between a girl with low self-esteem and a girl with a strong sense of herself and her abilities. Girls feel good about themselves when they can do well in school – especially in these subjects. Sometimes girls have difficulty because of the way that these subjects are taught. Most teachers teach math and science by stressing logic and abstraction. Both of these abilities are more suited to the male brain. While some girls do well in this kind of learning, others are at a disadvantage. This doesn't mean that most girls can't do math and science. It does mean that it has to be presented in the way that girls learn.

> "I used to like math," says Michelle. "But now I don't. Even when Mr. Green tries to help me I still don't understand it. He gets impatient with me, like I'm supposed to know it and I'm wasting his time. I feel really stupid and I just give up."

When I was young I had difficulty in math. I had a tutor in high school so that I could get through it. He was a reluctant tutor, and I ended up passing not so much because of an increase in skill but because of fear and intimidation. Things always seem to come full circle, so it was only natural that when I moved from teaching elementary school to high school, the subject that I was offered just happened to be math, for grades eight and nine. While I never became a good mathematician, I knew how to address the pitfalls that my students would face. Many years before I learned that there was such a thing as gender differences, I was already telling stories about x's and y's.

Giving Girls Feedback They Can Hear

Girls today face the future under a lot more pressure than we did. Along with becoming sexy wives and perfect mothers, both thin and beautiful, they also have to have a successful career. This means having good enough marks to get into university and competing in the job market at a time when jobs are scarce. Because we want them to succeed (we always want the best for them), we give them feedback and encouragement and try to help them with homework and projects even when they are still in elementary school. Sometimes we inadvertently increase the pressure on them because we give them feedback in a way that they can't hear.

As chapter 1 demonstrated, women and men speak and hear in different ways. There is no problem when we are bicultural, or familiar with these different communication rituals. We run into trouble, however, when we are not aware that we are speaking different languages, and make the assumption that what the other person said is what we think it means. It is relatively easy to connect with girls by helping them with their personal issues because we can communicate with them in a familiar female style. But when we try to give them academic (or sports) encouragement, we lose them because we begin to speak to them in "male."

Deborah Tannen writes in *Talking from 9 to 5* about communication differences in the workplace which can easily be applied to girls' experiences in school. Tannen tells the story of Amy, a manager who has to tell her male employee that his report was inadequate and that he has to do it again. "When Amy met with Donald," writes Tannen, "she made sure to soften the blow by beginning with praise, telling him everything about his report that was good. Then she went on to explain what was lacking and what needed to be done to make it acceptable." When the revised report was placed on her desk, it became evident that Donald had heard the praise but not the criticism. In order for him to hear the criticism, Amy would have to have been more direct.[13]

We give girls feedback in a manner that would have been more appropriate for Donald. We don't acknowledge what they have already done, but place the emphasis on what we think they should do. Because this is not how girls communicate, it makes them feel criticized personally, and makes them feel that their efforts go unacknowledged and unseen.

> "I worked so hard to do my project," says Carol, "and then my mom says to me 'Didn't you see those spelling

mistakes?' It makes me feel like everything I just did didn't count. It wasn't important."

"I leave my projects on the kitchen table when I go to bed at night," says Erin. "In the morning, my parents have already corrected it and have left me comments. I just want them to tell me that I did a good job."

"My father says that I should do more than the teacher asks," says Jodi. "I tell him that the other kids won't do extra – but he says that's how people get ahead. All I want is for him to tell me that he really liked what I already did."

We need to take a lesson from Amy when we give girls feedback. We need to first acknowledge what they have already done. Then we need to offer (not tell them) any changes that we think they might (not should) make.

"I want my mom and dad to tell me what they liked," says Erin. "I want them to tell me that they know I worked really hard."

"I want them to tell me that they know I worked hard," says Carol, "and that they think my ideas are really good. Then ask me if I want to make corrections, or if I want you to tell me where the mistakes are." ·

Girls need feedback that is specific. Words such as like, good, and interesting are *garbage can* words – they hold a lot, but don't have very much value. Knowing that we are praising something specific about what they have done helps them own their achievements. It also helps them learn from their mistakes.

Making the Transition to High School

The transition to high school (or junior high or middle school) can be difficult. The elementary schools are more suited to the way that girls learn. They are smaller and foster more intimacy and connection. Elementary school provides girls with the opportunity to work more cooperatively, which is the best way that most girls learn. Girls have the same teacher throughout the year. The same kids are in their class. While this may have some drawbacks, especially if they don't get along with the teacher, the faces do remain the same and the teacher does get to know a whole lot more about them – besides how they do in school.

One of the biggest fears that seventh grade girls voice is the transition to high school. Most high schools are huge. Girls now have different teachers. The interaction is more impersonal. One high school guidance counselor told me that she has a case load of 500 students. It's amazing that she can know anything about them – let alone recognize them when she sees them in the hall. Girls are often afraid that they won't know anyone and will end up all alone, because not all the same students are together in all of their classes. And even though they are excited at making new friends, they are also afraid of losing the ones they had before.

Sometimes it helps girls if they can visit the high school ahead of time and become familiar with the different routine. They need to know where the bathroom is before they need to use it and where the cafeteria is if they are going to have lunch in school. It is also most helpful when schools can set up a buddy system – where seventh grade girls can pair up with older girls. Then girls know at least one familiar face in the new place.

▶ Strategies to Consider

- Be specific in your feedback. Remember that words such as good, nice, interesting, are *garbage can* words. Let her know what makes things good, or nice or interesting. Let her know why you are suggesting changes.

- Ask for permission to make corrections. Girls need to know that their work belongs to them and that we respect their boundaries.

- Avoid sweeping generalizations. Girls at this stage of development are very concrete. They take what we say literally and can't see that there are any other options. Statements such as "you can be anything you want to be" don't encourage them. They make them feel pressured, because there is no option for the "don't want to be."

- Help her identify how she learns. We don't all learn the same way. Some of us are visually oriented and some auditory. Some of us are kinesthetic – we feel things in our body. Some of us are more concrete than others. Most of us are contextual. We need to frame things in terms of a story.

- Examine your motives. How do you see success? Ask yourself why you want her to be successful. Sometimes we try to live our own lives, or satisfy our own *shoulds* through the girls in our lives.

- Take her complaints seriously. Validate her feelings and experiences. Sometimes we try to explain them away. Later, I will talk about advocating for girls in the schools.

- Share yourself and your experiences. Yes, here it is again.

NOTES

1   Michael Hutchison. *The Anatomy of Sex and Power: An Investigation of Mind-Body Politics*. New York: William Morrow, 1990, p. 168.
2   Anne Moir and David Jessel. *Brain Sex: The Real Difference between Men and Women*. New York: Bantam Doubleday Dell, 1991, p. 62.
3   Myra Sadker and David Sadker. *Failing at Fairness: How Our Schools Cheat Girls*. New York: Simon & Schuster, 1994, pp. 5-8, 55.
4   Sadker and Sadker.
5   Sadker and Sadker.
6   Peggy Orenstein in association with the American Association of University Women. *SchoolGirls: Young Women, Self-Esteem and the Confidence Gap*. New York: Doubleday, 1994, p. 7.

7   Sadker and Sadker.

8   Sadker and Sadker.

9   Orenstein.

10 Sadker and Sadker.

11 The American Association of University Women Educational Foundation. *The AAUW Report: How Schools Shortchange Girls*. Washington, DC: The AAUW Educational Foundation and National Education Association, 1992, p. 28.

12 Heather Featherstone. "Girls' Math Achievement: What We Do and Don't Know." *The Harvard Education Letter*, January 1986, pp. 1-5.

13 Deborah Tannen. *Talking from 9 to 5: How Men's and Women's Conversational Styles Affect Who Gets Heard, Who Gets Credit and What Gets Done at Work*. New York: William Morrow, 1994, pp. 21-22.

16

Bullying and Harassment

At a grade seven workshop that I was facilitating, I asked for volunteers to role-play how they would deal with teasing and bullying. I chose "shoes" as a topic that would be neutral enough so that the girls playing victims would not end up feeling personally hurt by the "bullies." In each role-playing situation, the girls who were the "bullies" demonstrated the exquisite cruelty that girls inflict upon one another. They curled their lips and sneered. Their voices were contemptuous and taunting. Their body language was menacing. It took tremendous effort by the "victims" and support from the group for them not to collapse. Even I began to feel inadequate and convinced that I needed a more stylish and acceptable pair of shoes.

Bullying is one of the most frequent and difficult situations that students have to deal with in school today. An incident of bullying takes place once every seven minutes. It usually lasts about thirty-seven seconds. Its emotional effects can last a much longer time for the victim – and for others who witness the bullying. Its physical effects can be deadly.[1]

Bullying is intentional behavior. It doesn't occur because two people just happen to have a misunderstanding. Bullies seek power by hurting the other person. Boys bully other boys and bully girls to elevate their own status and increase their sense of adequacy. Girls bully girls whom they see as a threat to their relationships with other girls and to their relationships with boyfriends. Sometimes there is not a clear-cut line between who is a bully and who is a victim. When one sixth grade girl came to the group I was co-facilitating, crying that she was being picked on by the other girls, we spent the session on conflict resolution and communication skills. Although we thought the issue was resolved, the next week the same girl was tormenting someone else.

Physical bullying usually involves boys, although there is a growing number of girls. They kick and hit the victim and/or take and damage the victim's property. These bullies become more aggressive as they get older. Both girls and boys engage in verbal bullying or teasing and name-calling in order to hurt and humiliate others.

> "I used to play touch and tackle football in fifth grade," says twelve-year-old Brittany. "They used to make it touch for the girls and tackle for the boys. We could tackle them, but they could only touch us. The boys used to call us whale and wall and things like that."

Bullies emphasize whatever makes the victim different from his or her peers and use insults and racist comments. When boys tease each other their aggression takes the form of misogynist and homophobic taunts such as "fag," "wuss," and "girl." Girls focus on body size and personal characteristics.

> "I think that I am way too skinny," says eleven-year-old Marcie. "All my friends and lots of other people tease me about it. They also tease me because I have really big feet but I can't help it. They really hurt me."

Relational bullying is most often done by girls who exclude other girls from their peer groups, spread nasty rumors and tell secrets about them, tease them and frame them and set them up for punishment. This kind of bullying is devastating to girls who are rejected from their peer groups at the time that they need them the most.

> "Why do girls exclude other girls when we know it just hurts each other?" asks twelve-year-old Sarah during a discussion about bullying.

Girls who are being bullied often become reluctant to come to school, or to walk there and back all alone. They have headaches, stomach aches, and other bodily symptoms. They show signs of depression such as low energy, difficulty in sleeping, and eating too much or too little. They don't want to talk about what's happening in school, and if they do they don't want parental or teacher intervention because they are afraid of being singled out and being made subject to worse treatment.[2]

> "What do you do," asked Katrina, "when you constantly get called names like fat, but you don't want to tell because you think it's going to happen even more?"

Dealing with bullying is difficult. Because we adults don't know what to do, we often hide behind creative denial. We tell the boys to fight back and the girls to walk away. We tell girls and boys to stop being so sensitive. We normalize teasing by telling them that this is what they have to expect from life.

> "The boys call us pigs and cows and fat," complains ten-year-old Fiona. "When we tell the teacher, she says they do this because they like us."

When we talk about zero tolerance in our schools but don't enforce it, we teach students that no one will stand up for them. We need to work together with teachers, students, support staff and school administration to encourage students to report bullies and to provide them with safety when they do. This means guaranteeing students that the bullying will stop; that it will be stopped in such a way that no one knows who reported it; and that the bully will be treated firmly but with understanding.[3] If the adults don't follow up with action, then the students will feel not only unsafe but also betrayed.

Although it is hard for us as individuals to stop bullying behavior in the school, there are steps we can take to support our girls. We can help them build friendship connections and encourage them to participate in activities that will reduce the isolation that makes them vulnerable. We also help girls name the behavior, validate their feelings, ensure them that they have a right to safety, and teach them skills and techniques for dealing with bullying situations.

Sexual Harassment

Sexual harassment is a form of bullying. It includes unwanted touching, verbal comments and name-calling; the spreading of sexual rumors, gestures, jokes or cartoons, and notes; and conversations that are too personal. The term was coined during the mid-1970s by a group of Cornell University women who were looking for a way to describe the treatment of a campus employee who had been refused repeated requests to be transferred away from a colleague who was hounding her. Today, the existence of sexual harassment is recognized in all levels of education as well as in the workplace.[4]

Sexual Harassment Begins in Elementary School

It's harder to be a kid today than when we were growing up. Kids today are constantly being exposed to raw, explicit sexual imagery from sources as diverse as prime time television, pop music, video games, movies, billboard advertising, the Internet and talk radio. They are also exposed to more violence. Sexual harassment is learned at an early age. In elementary school, girls are called "sluts," "whores" (or "hos"), "cunts" and "bitches" by boys who pinch their breasts, lift their skirts and thrust their hands between girls' legs.

> "Marcy and I play soccer," says eleven-year-old Gina. "Last year when we were in fifth grade, all the fifth grade boys played soccer on the field and that's when we would get called names. They called us whores and fucking bitches. They didn't have any reason to call us that. If we take the ball we're bitches. Or if a girl checks them or if she scores, then they call her a fucking whore."

> "There is this boy in my drama class," says thirteen-year-old Michelle. "He came up to me and told me to give him a blow job. He said if I didn't he would tell all his friends that I did."

We are often tempted to view this behavior as normal. We say boys will be boys. When we look at their actions in a broader context, we are able to place this behavior at the beginning of a continuum of violence that begins in elementary school with teasing and grabbing, and can later escalate into date rape and physical abuse. We see in the newspapers daily that women at the farthest extreme of this continuum end up dead.

In *Hostile Hallways*, a study commissioned by the American Association of University Women Educational Foundation, researchers found that 81 percent of students (both boys and girls) in eighth through eleventh grades have experienced sexual harassment.[5] When the Wellesley College Center for Research on Women and the National Organization for Women (NOW) Legal Defense Fund analyzed responses to a reader survey in *Seventeen* magazine, they found that 89 percent of girls aged nine to nineteen experienced sexual harassment in their schools. Eighty-nine percent reported inappropriate sexual comments, gestures and looks, and 83 percent had been touched, pinched or grabbed. Forty percent said that these incidents occurred daily.[6]

It's not only boys who sexually harass girls. In a grade seven group, Cari described how her teacher responded to her when she wanted to do her project with two boys who were her friends.

> "He told me that I couldn't work with them," said Cari. "He said when girls were developing the way that I was, they got the boys all excited and then they couldn't work."

> "Mr. Taylor always talks like that," confirmed her friend Michelle. "He says that he likes to teach seventh grade because the kids are developing. And then he looks at our breasts and says, 'And some of you are developing a lot more than others.'"

When boys and men make comments about girls' bodies, girls come to feel that their bodies are not their own. In 1949, Simone de Beauvoir wrote in *The Second Sex*:

> The young woman feels her body is getting away from her, it is no longer the straightforward expression of her individuality; at the same time she becomes for others a thing; on the street men follow her with their eyes and comment on her body. She would like to be invisible; it frightens her to become flesh and show her flesh.[7]

Years later it seems that not very much is different. At a time when girls are most vulnerable because of the many changes that are happening to them, sexual harassment and objectification intensify the process by which they disconnect from their bodies and thus from themselves.

Sometimes girls push back. They call the boys names in return. While such behavior is condoned in boys it is rarely accepted in girls. When the harasser is a person in power, such as a teacher, the girls often don't have anywhere to go. They don't tell their parents because they are afraid that they will be singled out later on. When harassment is not recognized in the schools and when girls don't have an outlet and validation for their feelings, they turn the harassment against themselves.[8] Along with the shame and loathing that they feel for their bodies, many girls also feel fat.

> "When Mr. Taylor told me why I couldn't do my project with the boys," says Cari, "I felt like there was something wrong with me. I felt really fat."

Sexual Harassment Escalates in High School

Sexual harassment that is not stopped at the beginning of the continuum often escalates in high school. Girls often can't walk down the hall without being grabbed and groped. They don't feel safe when they participate in class.

> "I'm in ninth grade," says Terri. "In one of my classes there are a few boys who pick on me. They make fun of my breasts and repeatedly slam the desk into my back and then ask if I am going to cry."

Sexual harassment puts girls at physical risk. In one study, 38 percent of the women who reported date rape were between the ages of fourteen and seventeen.[9] Sexual harassment and date rape stem from the same attitudes – that men and boys have a right to control women and girls. When sexual harassment enters the dating scene, many girls don't even know when they have been raped.[10]

When girls are victims of sexual harassment in high school, it affects their self-esteem and interferes with their performance in school. In order to avoid the behaviors, girls stop participating in class discussions so as not to call attention to themselves. They don't take courses if certain boys are in them. They skip classes so that they won't have to be subjected to antifemale remarks or taunting behavior. Sometimes when the harassment gets really bad, girls feel that they have no option but to change schools.[11]

Parent Power

Parents don't often hear about the harassment. Sometimes girls keep silent because they are afraid they won't be believed. Sometimes girls feel they should be able to fight their battles on their own, or that the harassment is a result of something they have done. Sometimes their daughters won't tell them because they are afraid that the repercussions will be even worse if their parents interfere. When parents do find out, they get angry and wonder what to do next.

> "I haven't heard any of this until today – especially the vicious name-calling," says Cari's mom. "It really upsets me. I can remember being that age and being called a prostitute and going home and telling my mother. I remember asking my mother what a prostitute was. Kids were just trying the words out to bug each other, but it wasn't really in an intimidating way. This sounds really intimidating and more frequent."
>
> "It really bothered me when I heard Brittany talk about what's going on," says June. "It looks like boys start using these tactics whenever girls excel at something they think they should be better at. The girls are targets whenever they are out there. Why is there nobody in the school willing to support the girls?"

When parents approach the school they are sometimes met with cooperation. These are usually schools in which a sexual harassment policy is in place, and there is no tolerance for violence of any kind. Many schools and school boards are like ostriches, however, and prefer to keep their heads in the sand. They are very big at promoting self-esteem and healthy classrooms, but won't look at the harassment issue – which undermines all their other efforts.

Susan Strauss wrote the state harassment-prevention curriculum for Minnesota, which is used by the AAUW and is a model for other states. She says that parents who complain about sexual harassment in the schools often have to deal with denial, apathy and hostility from the school boards. They often have to deal with lack of community support.[12] If you try to address sexual harassment, you run the risk of ridicule when the schools are not ready to listen to what you have to say. If you decide to keep silent, you let your daughters down because you don't stand up on their behalf.

Sometimes addressing sexual harassment is systemic. Teachers may be willing to address it; but when the parents of boys complain, the teachers don't receive backing from the administration, or the administration doesn't receive backing from the boards.

It is becoming harder now for schools to minimize or ignore sexual harassment. On May 24, 1999, in a case called *Aurelia Davis v Monroe County Board of Education*, the Supreme Court ruled 5 to 4 that any school receiving federal money can face a sex-discrimination suit under Title IX for failing to intervene energetically enough when a student complains of sexual harassment by another student. To avoid a lawsuit, schools must take complaints seriously and must show that they have stopped, or have tried to stop, the harassment.[13]

▶ *Strategies to Consider*

- Take her concerns seriously.
- Help her put a name to what's going on. This makes it real.
- Let her know that bullying is hurtful and that she has a right to be safe when she goes to school. Let her know that in the adult world sexual harassment is against the law. This helps validate her concerns.

- Encourage details. What do people call you? What do they do? Talking about bullying or sexual harassment in a safe atmosphere helps defuse the power of the words and helps her get rid of the shame.

- Describe bullying and/or sexual harassment as an issue of power. Girls need to know that it has nothing to do with their adequacy as a friend or how they look.

- Talk about how you are going to deal with her complaints. Can she tell the principal herself? What kind of support does she need? What kind of support will you need?

- She may not want you to intercede, but it's your job to protect her. If you don't say anything, you are tacitly conspiring with the offender. Secrets that protect people who victimize you can turn against you the longer they are kept inside.

- Build allies with other parents. The more voices there are, the more it becomes a school problem and not an individual one.

- Lobby for conflict resolution and communication skills to be taught in the early grades.

- Help her fight back. Bullies usually stop if we don't react to the content of what they are saying. Our reaction is what fuels their aggression. Review the section on defensive behavior in chapter 8 and help her stand up to the bully:

  - Role-play the "bully" and the "victim."

  - Each time the bully says something, have the victim repeat, "Stop. I don't like what you are saying." "Stop. I don't like what you are saying." (It's tempting to respond to the content, so the victim may need additional support.) Continue until the bully stops. Switch roles and do it again. If she gets scared, let her know that she can walk away whenever she wants.

Time Out for Yourself

It's hard to read about sexual harassment. The language is strong and it's painful to think that the girls we love can be at risk of any kind of violence, or that these things happen in our schools. Yet again and again studies and stories tell us that these things do happen.

We may think that these kinds of things didn't happen when we were growing up but in fact they did. The difference was that these incidents were not so overt, and that we didn't have the language to describe what was going on.

> "When I first heard about sexual harassment in the schools, I was very shocked," says Carly. "Then I sat back and thought about it and remembered the boys in seventh grade telling me that they wanted to screw me. I didn't have a clue what they meant."

Think back to your own puberty, adolescence, and even adulthood:

- Can you remember a time when a boy or man made any comment about your body that made you uncomfortable?

- Can you remember a time when a boy or man made a sexual suggestion to you that made you feel uncomfortable, or touched your breasts, crotch or buttocks, even in a supposedly playful manner?

- How did that make you feel?

- How did you handle the situation?

- What do you wish that you could have said?

Notes

1   Gesele Lajoie, Alyson McLellan and Cindi Seddon. *Take Action against Bullying*. Coquitlam, BC: Bully Beware Productions, 1997.

2   Lajoie et al.

3   Lajoie et al.

4   Cynthia Gorney. "Teaching Johnny the Appropriate Way to Flirt," *New York Times Magazine*, June 13, 1999.

5   American Association of University Women Education Foundation. *Hostile Hallways: The AAUW Survey on Sexual Harassment in America's Schools.* Researched by Harris/Scholastic Research, a division of Louis Harris and Associates in partnership with Scholastic, Inc. Washington, DC: AAUW Educational Foundation, 1993, p. 12.

6   Nan Stein, Nancy L. Marshall and Linda R. Tropp. *Secrets in Public: Sexual Harassment in Our Schools*. Wellesley, MA: Center for Research on Women, Wellesley College, and the NOW Legal Defense and Education Fund, 1993, p. 7.

7   Simone de Beauvoir, *The Second Sex* (2nd ed., H.M. Parshley, trans.). New York: Vintage Books, 1972, p. 346.

8   June Larkin, Carla Rice and Vanessa Russel, "Slipping through the Cracks: Sexual Harassment, Eating Problems and the Problem of Embodiment," in *Eating Disorders: Journal of Treatment and Prevention*, Vol. 4, No. 1 (Spring 1996), p. 9.

9   Barrie Levy, ed. *Dating Violence: Young Women in Danger*. Seattle: The Seal Press, 1991.

10 June Larkin. *Sexual Harassment: High School Girls Speak Out*. Toronto: Second Story Press, 1994, pp. 94-111.

11 Larking.

12 Susan Strauss. *Sexual Harassment and Teens: A Program for Positive Change*, Minneapolis, MN: Free Spirit Publishing, 1988.

13 Gorney.

17

⁂

Continuing
the Journey

In a grade six group, the girls are drawing pictures. They are
trying to depict what it is like to be a girl today. Eleven-year-
old Cody draws a garden. "Girls are like flowers," she explains.
She describes the different girls in her class and adds, "There are
all kinds of girls. They come in all sizes and colors and shapes."

Before adolescence, girls may indeed remind us of flowers.
They grow strong and vibrant in the well-nourished soil of childhood. They turn their faces to the sun. In the sheltered environment
of elementary school, most girls feel good about themselves and their
abilities. Maturing faster than boys, they are ready for math and
reading earlier and develop better control of their small motor skills,
which enable them to write. The emphasis on cooperation, communication and learning in small groups is consistent with their
female culture. They are rewarded for their skills at social interaction. Girls flourish here despite the fact that more attention is paid
to the boys in the classroom.

As girls approach adolescence, the very skills and qualities that
make them feel good about themselves suddenly betray them. Girls

develop their identity (sense of self) in the context of their relationships, but the male culture views closeness in negative terms – placing a higher value on independence and individuality. Girls' emphasis on connection is reframed by society as neediness and dependence. Their interdependence is interpreted as indecision, as constantly needing someone else's approval, and not being able to make up their minds.

Girls soon come to believe that there is something wrong with them, that what they say and how they say it has no value. They begin to doubt themselves and their abilities. They reinvent themselves to fit into the male culture by repressing those parts of themselves that are deemed unacceptable. Looking outside themselves for definition, they erect barriers between their true selves and the socially accepted persona that they feel the need to create. When they stop speaking about what they really feel and try instead to please others, the boundary between what they know to be true and what they project outward slowly becomes blurred. Girls lose their own ability to tell the difference between what they feel inside and what they project.

While most are hardy and can withstand difficult conditions, just like flowers they tend to wither and wilt when they are transplanted into hostile soil, and we run the risk that their very spirits will die.

At the time when our culture is pressuring girls to disconnect from their selves, the media instructs them that there is something wrong with their bodies. The media bombards girls with messages that fat is bad, that everyone wants to be thin, and that they can achieve an "ideal" body if only they try hard enough. Girls compare themselves to what they see on television and in magazines. The bodies that are held out to girls as models are often products of technology. To achieve anything resembling them exacts a high price in terms of a girl's health.

Girls who are going through puberty and dealing with the attendant weight gain and increase in body fat look at their changing bodies and feel shame instead of excitement. Associating the weight gain that occurs in puberty with the messages broadcast by the greater culture, they try to deal with their discomfort over the changes in their lives by focusing on their bodies. They begin to feel fat.

It's hard to grow up female today without ever feeling fat. Fat has become a dirty word in our culture, and girls use it to insult each other. They also use it as a way of redirecting their distress against themselves. When girls have no safe place to talk about what is real, when they can't express their feelings directly, many encode them in the language of fat. Girls feel fat when they are happy. They feel fat when they are sad. They feel fat when they are disappointed or angry or lonely or any of a myriad of feelings that they can't easily express. Girls feel fat when they doubt themselves and their opinions and have no context for the changes that are taking place in their lives.

The language of fat serves for a very large number of girls as a misdirected means of expression – one that affects their self-esteem. For others, it may extend into obsessive behaviors centered around food and weight. Anorexia, bulimia, compulsive eating and other obsessive behaviors may develop out of this preoccupation. When carried to an extreme, eating disorders can result in real medical risk.

Eating disorders are the third greatest health risk to girls today. In our panic to stop them we focus on the behaviors instead of addressing what they really mean. If we wish to prevent girls from becoming entrapped by the preoccupation with food and weight, then we need to teach them how to express their feelings directly and how to deal with the stresses in their lives without turning these against themselves. We can do this by helping girls recognize when they feel fat, and by encouraging them to talk about the real issues that lie underneath. We need to validate their feelings and provide them with language to describe those experiences so that they understand why they feel the way they do.

We're exposed to the same societal influences and pressure from the media that our girls experience. We, too, have learned to speak in the language of fat. We, too, try to gain control over our lives by trying to control the size of our bodies. We, too, need to look at our relationship with food and weight and re-examine our attitudes toward people whom we call fat. Many of us go on diets whenever we are under stress. We eat our way through our crises, binge, purge or fast and count our grams of fat with the same precision as pharmacists dispensing life-saving drugs. While we don't need to give up our coping mechanisms or resolve our uneasy relationships with food right away, we need to become aware of and curious about our own behavior and attitudes – because we pass them along to girls.

The best way that we can help girls through adolescence is to imagine them as flowers and cultivate them like gardeners. We need to nurture them to keep their spirits alive. If we can trust ourselves and each other, work together, and remain connected to the girls in our lives, we can help them grow strong and take their rightful places in the world.

Maintaining Our Connections through Adolescence

As mothers we are the primary role models for our girls as they grow up. The most important people in their lives – at least for a while. They confide in us when they are younger, but by the time they reach high school, girls become reticent to reveal themselves to us as they transfer their interdependence to their friends. Girls look to their peer group for guidance and approval. They experiment with new behaviors and values and try to present an image of themselves as cool. When girls move us out of center stage it doesn't mean they are no longer interested in us. It means that our relationship is in the process of being redefined.

We need to ignore the societal myth that girls must separate from us in order to create a life of their own. When girls become adolescents they need their connection with us to remain strong more than ever. Girls look to us to help them sort out what is expected of them and figure out what they should be like. They need us to act as a sounding board as they try on different attitudes and stances to see which ones will fit. We can help girls make sense of things so they can decide for themselves what is right. We have to take care, however, that we don't give in to the pressure to make them fit into the culture because by doing so we reinforce the very same conditions that cause them to feel fat.

Instead of shooting down their ideas (no matter how outrageous they may seem), we can be curious about the process that they go through to arrive at their opinions, and listen to what these mean to them. We can praise girls when they make healthy decisions and tell them we admire how they handle themselves. Giving girls specific feedback offers them a vision of themselves that goes beyond pretty and nice.

As girls ride the waves of adolescent hormones their feelings change very quickly and tend to be quite intense. At this stage of their development, girls have difficulty seeing beyond the immediate situation. They also think that if they *feel* something, then it is true. This intensity makes their problems seem very powerful to them. Girls at this time constantly test us to see if we are strong enough to handle their problems. They are afraid that we will become hysterical, fall apart or be otherwise overwhelmed. Girls need us to provide them with consistency and perspective. When we take their crises and failures personally, we are not able to give them that support. When we react with intensity of our own, they stop sharing things with us – because they don't want to take care of our feelings in addition to trying to deal with their own.

Girls watch us to see how we negotiate our own relationships. They look to see if we give away our power or if we stand up for ourselves. It's painful for them to have a mother or a female mentor who lets herself be treated with disrespect, one who cannot therefore respect herself. When this happens girls make a decision that they won't be like us. When we don't model a healthy way of being in charge of our lives, then girls will look to the male model and try to be independent, to not need anyone. And in giving up their connections with others, they lose their connection with themselves.

Girls respond to us when they feel connected to us. The greatest gift that we can give them is our honesty and willingness to be real. Girls need us to listen to them with our hearts instead of always with our heads. They need us to talk *to* them instead of *at* them. They need us to validate their feelings and actions instead of telling them what to do. This means that we must be able to step out of the protection of our roles as mothers (and other mentors) and risk being ourselves.

They don't need us to be perfect or together or to have all the answers or to always be right. When they can see our own struggles and failings, it gives them permission to engage in their struggles and to risk having failings of their own. When girls see that we can embrace the messiness that goes along with being human and still feel good about ourselves, it gives them the strength to resist society's one-dimensional model of perfection and helps them hang on to their sense of self.

It's sometimes hard to stay open and receptive when girls go through adolescence. Some girls make it through the changes without any glitches, but others kick up a storm. One day their energy puts them on top of the world, and we all bask in their reflected joy and good will. The next day they are crying inconsolably. They slam the door and tell us we don't understand them. We throw up our hands in frustration and just hope that they will come home all right. When girls are irritable, moody and inconsolable, it's hard not to take it personally, to understand that their angst is probably not even about us and that they are probably dealing with problems around school or friends. On the one hand, girls want to be close to us. On the other, they challenge everything we say. There's a cartoon on my wall of a mother and teenage daughter, with the mother asking, "Why don't you leave now, when you know everything?" That seems to say it all.

Girls of this age want us to approve of everything that they are doing. When we don't, they get angry and tell us that we couldn't possibly understand. While we would like to be supportive, our frame of reference is different from theirs and so some of the things that they talk about make us uncomfortable and some of their behavior seems pretty weird. We want to respect their need to establish their own identity, but we also know that short skirts, cut-off tops, baggy or torn clothes, long purple hair, shaved heads, nose rings and/or body piercing would cause us to die of embarrassment if we had to present ourselves in public that way.

We have to ask ourselves what it is about the adolescent cultural badges that make us object to them. We need to examine our own *shoulds* and our own tapes. We need to choose our battles wisely and to limit our objections according to the degree of harm their behavior might do. There is a vast difference between allowing girls to get a fourth hole pierced in their ear – when they tell us that that's what the other girls do – and letting them serve alcohol at a teenage party.

Girls need limits and boundaries to ensure their safety and to help them take responsibility for themselves. It's often hard for us to find a balance between being too controlling in our attempts to protect girls, and too permissive because we are afraid of their anger. It's hard not to yield to their pressure that everyone is doing "it" and they don't want to be different from their friends. We need to be clear about who we are and what is important to us. No matter how much we want to support girls, we need to remember who is the adult and who is the child.

Girls respond best when they know that we love them and that we also mean what we say. We need to know who their friends are and how girls spend their free time. We need them to call home to check in with us and to let us know when they are late. We need to have input in their activities and in the time that they spend with their friends. This means saying no to overnighters when we feel that they are getting out of hand. Because our efforts are often met with objection, we need to keep the lines of communication open and learn to fight fair. Because most of us see disagreement as rejection, we have to learn to separate the behavior from the worth of the person involved, and take responsibility for ourselves.

While as mothers we want the best for our girls, we have to recognize that we can't do it all alone. Families are under tremendous pressure today. Things have changed since the 1950s, when one salary could support a family of four. In today's global economy, a few people have a lot of money while most of us have to do with less than enough. We work longer hours today and live under the threat that our jobs won't be here tomorrow, or that we will have to take pay cuts to enable our companies to survive.

Time has also become a scarce commodity. As women we are most often the ones responsible for cooking, cleaning and child-rearing – on top of the work that we do outside our homes. Many of us don't live in the same communities or cities that we grew up in so we don't have families that we can fall back on for support. Most days not only is it difficult to make time for the girls in our lives, we don't have time for ourselves.

Building Different Kinds of Support

We have to recognize, no matter how painful, that there might be times when we cannot be there in the way that girls need us because of other stresses in our lives. Sometimes – regardless of what we try to give them – girls cannot take it in. Sometimes our relationships can go through such turbulent times that we reach an impasse and have to call time out. We need to accept that at certain times and in certain situations, girls need a different kind of support.

Girls need a mentor – someone they can have a less emo-tionally charged relationship with, someone who doesn't see them as a reflection of themselves. They need someone to talk to who can validate their feelings and help them understand the changes in their lives without worrying how they present themselves and what they are going to do. Girls need someone who can help them sort out their relationship with their mothers (and fathers) so that they can keep the connection with them alive. When life becomes too full of unresolved conflict, girls need an outsider who can see them – and help them see themselves – in a more positive light. Having an anchor when times are difficult often makes the dif-ference between girls being able to hold their head above water or drowning emotionally.

There is no one model for a mentor. She can be an older cousin, a friend of the family, a teacher, school nurse, swimming instructor or coach, or the neighbor next door. A mentor can be someone with whom girls can develop a lasting relationship. She can also be someone who happens to be there just at the right time and right place. When I was in elementary school the school librarian tossed me a self-saver when she introduced me to the world of books. As I went through adolescence and my relationship with my mother became a battleground, I was fortunate to have an aunt who lived downstairs from me, and the mother of a good friend who lived down the street.

One of the most powerful kinds of support for girls during adolescence is the kind that comes from groups. Like the consciousness raising groups that women went to in the seventies, girls' groups can help them put language to the changes that are happening to them in adolescence. This lets them know that they are not alone in how they feel. In the groups that I've developed and facilitated, we encourage girls to express their feelings and provide them with a context for their concerns. The group setting gives girls an opportunity to be listened to and taken seriously, something that most girls rarely experience and which they badly need. Girls look forward to each session and make changes in how they see themselves. Just thinking about what they are going to say each week helps them take their focus off other people and redirect it to themselves.

Groups can allow girls to try out new behavior and support them as they practice it in their lives. They can teach girls good communication and conflict resolution skills, so that they can sustain honest relationships with one another and hold back the tyranny of kind and nice. They can help girls hold on to and validate their female culture, and so feel good about themselves. They can help girls express themselves directly so that they don't have to feel fat.

Claiming Girls' Space in the World

While we need to empower girls on an individual basis, we also need to make sure they claim their space in the world. This means ensuring that female culture – their ideas, opinions and ways of doing things – is a part of the society in which we live. A while ago I participated in a conference called "Our Issues, Our Lives." The conference was organized by the young women in the tenth grade of one secondary school, along with their dedicated vice-principal and guidance counselors. One hundred and fifty participants came from surrounding schools. Over the two days of the conference they attended workshops, met women from a wide range of occupations and professions, watched a local female comic and several student skits, and listened to an address by a prominent politician – a role model herself.

The young women generated incredible energy at the conference. McDonald's provided the food. On the second day, I asked one young woman if she was becoming exhausted by this point. "Oh no," she said to me, surprised at the question. "They are speaking about what is in my heart." We need to provide girls with opportunities to have what's in their heart reflected back to them from our society. Events like this one demonstrate to girls that their concerns are important and, by extension, so are the girls themselves.

While it's not difficult to organize girls-only events, we need to prepare for the backlash that they create. Often when I advocate for resources for girls, I am asked "What about the boys?" There is no question that boys also need groups and resources to provide them with healthy modeling of what it is to be a man. We need to be clear, however, that we are not talking about an either/or situation and that these resources don't come at the expense of the girls. I am also asked if mixed groups would be better, so that boys can learn about girls. While mixed groups can offer girls and boys a chance to know each other better, they don't provide girls with the much needed opportunity to learn about themselves.

Girls need to see themselves reflected positively in the outside world. They need to see their issues included in the public agenda. They also need to be exposed to a range of female activities so that they understand how multifaceted the lives of women and girls can be. One way of broadening their experience is to participate in the "Take a Daughter to Work™ Day." This is an annual event that was started by *Ms.* magazine.[1] If there is no "Take a Daughter to Work ™ Day" in your community, you can start one. If you don't work outside your home, ask a friend who does to take your daughter to work. Some schools arrange for students to "shadow" someone in a profession or occupation that might interest them. While it is important to let girls know the opportunities that are available to them outside the home, it is also important that they recognize the value of the work that we do inside the home.

Our support for girls needs to extend beyond our personal relationships. Although the connections may not always be obvious to us, our self-esteem (or lack of it) and our personal growth are linked to social and political change. Girls can't flourish under conditions of inequality or unfairness. They can't feel good about themselves when they don't have a voice in our society – when the messages that they convey are not the right ones or are simply not heard.

We can support organizations such as the YWCA, the Girl Scouts and Girl Guides, Big Sisters, and Girls Incorporated, which are trying to bring about change. Girls Incorporated (formerly Girls Clubs of America) is a national youth organization that provides education programs to 350,000 girls in the United States between the ages of six and eighteen. Girls Inc. is participating in a long-term, nationwide media and education project called "Girls Re-Cast TV." Part of the campaign is an action kit for girls.[2] It raises issues such as "Do girls and women on TV look like you or anyone you know?" and provides information – including addresses for writing TV network bosses.

We can take whatever actions we as individuals are comfortable taking to try to create a more equitable world. We can write letters to advertisers and lobby politicians so that we can create more opportunities for girls and change how they are seen in the world. When we begin to wonder what power one voice has, we need to remember that advertisers are sensitive to consumers – advertisers like Calvin Klein will pull an ad because of public outcry. Politicians need public support to legitimize what they want to do. We can participate in parent action councils, or home-and-school associations, or our own professional associations, and fight for girls' rights for gender equity in education and for our schools to be safe and free of harassment. We can be active in our communities and elect politicians who will actively support our views.

Supporting Each Other: All For One and One for All

We have to acknowledge how hard it is to raise a daughter, or to work with girls, during this period in their lives. We need to seek out and leave ourselves open to support from other women and, whenever it is available, from men. The mothers I talked to and interviewed supported one another. They found that talking to each other let them know they were not alone in how they felt. They validated each other's right to get angry when girls pushed their buttons. They helped each other set limits, and let each other know when they were being too wimpy or too hard. Other women give us perspective – because their experience is similar to ours. Women who have already lived through girls' puberty (and adolescence) let us know that it eventually comes to an end and that all concerned do survive it.

As the stresses and strains of our lives as mothers (and fathers) spill over into the schools, more and more demands are made on teachers, counselors, and school nurses to help support our girls. Living in a time of cutbacks, and as resources are becoming scarcer, it's difficult for us individually and as a society to deal with the burgeoning needs and the lack of public support. We have to recognize that as mothers and other mentors we can do more if we pool our resources than if we stand alone. We need to begin by speaking the same language, defining the same problems and working toward the same goals.

Some Words for the Road

Often when I do professional training with women, I simulate a girls' group, or what they like to call a "grungie group." The women sit in a circle. They remember the last time they felt fat and talk about what was underneath. The stories that the women tell are very personal. One woman is under tremendous pressure: she is trying to juggle full-time work with raising three kids. One woman has just broken up with her partner. She gets in touch with some of her anger and her grief. One woman is recovering from an illness. She recognizes how hard she is being on herself when she expects herself to do the same things in her period of recovery that she was able to do before.

When I ask for questions and feedback after the group has ended, a familiar dynamic surfaces. These competent, capable women suddenly begin to discount their own abilities, and begin to focus on mine instead. It is as if each time we undertake a new endeavor, we present ourselves like a computer with an empty harddrive. We cancel out all our previous experience. We delete our history and intuition, and give our power to somebody else.

We have to remember that as mothers and other mentors we are the experts. We may learn new skills as we guide girls through adolescence, but for the most part we draw upon resources that have already served us well. The mothers that I spoke to all had hopes for the future. What they wanted most was for their girls to find their voice, and to feel good about who they are.

> "I really hope that she speaks up for herself. I want her to be able to speak when she wants to speak, to be quiet when she wants to be quiet, and for that to be OK with her and with everybody else."

> "I would like her to be strong in how she feels about herself. To feel that she exists, that she is valuable, and that she is talented. It's sort of like an inner strength that you have that carries you through all different situations. I guess that tied to this is a strong voice. I want her to say what she wants. I want her to make demands of life. I want her to be able to say, 'This is what I want.'"

> "I want her to be well-rounded. I'd like her to go to college, but that's not the most important thing. I want her to feel good about herself and to have good friends and to have a balanced life."

I've envisioned this book as a kind of journey – one that has taken us through the world of girls. I've raised some issues that you might not have otherwise considered, and maybe taught you something about yourself that you didn't know before. I have provided a synthesis of much of the information about girls that is available and have included even more in the following resources section.

This kind of learning is a life-long process. While I hope that the skills and strategies I've given you are useful, I also hope that you will continue the journey long after you have put down this book. If I have succeeded in my task, this book may remain a valuable resource for you to consult – but I hope that you first learn to place your trust closer to home where it truly belongs: in yourself.

Notes

1   See Resources for additional information.
2   See Resources for additional information.

RESOURCES

Suggested
Readings and Videos

Gender and Female Development

The Girl Within. Emily Hancock. New York: Fawcett Columbine, 1989.

Meeting at the Crossroads: Women's Psychology and Girls' Development. Carol Gilligan and Lyn Mikel Brown. Cambridge: Harvard University Press, 1992.

Women's Growth in Connection: Writings from the Stone Center. Judith Jordan, Alexandra G. Kaplan, Jean Baker Miller, Irene P Stiver and Janet L. Surrey. New York: Guilford Press, 1991.

You Just Don't Understand: Women and Men in Conversation. Deborah Tannen. New York: Ballantine Books, 1990.

The Brain

Brain Sex: The Real Difference between Men and Women. Anne Moir and David Jessel. New York: Bantam Doubleday Dell, 1991.

Sex on the Brain: The Biological Differences between Men and Women. Deborah Blum. New York: Viking, 1997.

Eating Disorders and the Preoccupation with Food and Weight

Consuming Passions: Feminist Approaches to Weight Preoccupation and Eating Disorders. Catrina Brown and Karin Jasper, eds. Toronto: Second Story Press, 1993.

Coping with Eating Disorders (a book for adolescents). Barbara Moe. New York: Rosen Publishing Group, 1991.

Feminist Perspectives on Eating Disorders. Patricia Fallon, Melanie Katzman and Susan Wooley, eds. New York: Guilford Press, 1994.

Surviving an Eating Disorder: Strategies for Families and Friends. Michelle Siegel, Judith Brisman and Margot Weinshel. New York: HarperCollins, 1988.

Eating Disorder Prevention

Full of Ourselves: Advancing Girl Power, Leadership and Health: A Program Promoting the Healthy Development of Girls and the Prevention of Eating Disorders. Boston, MA: Harvard Eating Disorders Center.

Available from:
Harvard Eating Disorders Center
356 Boylston St.
Boston, MA 02116
617-236-7766

Just for Girls: A Group Program to Help Girls Navigate the Rocky Road through Adolescence and Avoid Pitfalls Such as Eating Disorders and the Preoccupation with Food and Weight. Sandra Susan Friedman. Vancouver, BC: Salal Books, 1999. (Contains blueprint for the program, plans for eighteen structured sessions, and twenty-five reproducible handouts.)

Available from:
Salal Books
#309, 101-1184 Denman Street
Vancouver, BC, Canada V6G 2M9
Telephone and Fax: (604) 689-8399
web site: www.salal.com
e-mail: salal@salal.net
Healthy Body Image: Teaching Kids to Eat and Love Their Bodies Too! Kathy J. Kater.

Available from:
Eating Disorders Awareness and Prevention, Inc. (EDAP)
603 Stewart Street, Suite 803
Seattle, WA 98101
Tel: (206) 382-3587
Fax: (206) 829-8501
(Toll free) 1-800-931-2237
web site: www.edap.org

Preventing Childhood Eating Problems: A Practical Positive Approach to Raising Children Free of Food and Weight Conflicts. Jane R. Hirschmann and Lela Zaphiropoulous. California: Gürze Books, 1993.

Preventing Eating Disorders: A Handbook of Interventions and Special Challenges. Niva Piran, Michael P. Levine and Catherine Steiner-Adair, eds. Philadelphia: Taylor and Francis, 1999.

Eating Disorder Information and Referral

American Anorexia/Bulimia Association (AABA)
293 Central Park West, Suite 1R
New York, NY 10024
(212) 501-8351

418 East 76th Street
New York, NY 10021
(212) 734-1114

Anorexia Nervosa and Related Eating Disorders, Inc. (ANRED)
P.O. Box 5102
Eugene, OR 97405
(503) 344-1144

Eating Disorders Awareness and Prevention, Inc. (EDAP)
603 Stewart Street, Suite 803
Seattle, WA 98101
Tel: (206) 382-3587
Fax: (206) 829-8501
(Toll free) 1-800-931-2237
web site: www.edap.org

Harvard Eating Disorders Center
356 Boylston Street
Boston, MA 02116
(617) 236-7766

National Association of Anorexia Nervosa and Associated Disorders (ANAD)
Highland Hospital
Highland Park, IL 60035
(708) 432-8000

National Center for Overcoming Overeating
P.O. Box 1257, Old Chelsea Station
New York, NY 10113-0920
(212) 875-0442

National Eating Disorder Information Centre (NEDIC)
CW 1, 304-200 Elizabeth Street
Toronto, ON M5G 2C4
Tel: (416) 340-4156
Fax: (416) 340-5888
web site: www.medic.on.ca

Parenting Girls

All That She Can Be: Helping Your Daughter Achieve Her Full Potential and Maintain Her Self-Esteem during the Critical Years of Adolescence. Dr. Carol J. Eagle and Carol Colman. New York: Simon & Schuster, 1993.

DADS AND DAUGHTERS (DADs)
PO Box 3458
Duluth, MN 55803
(Toll free) 1-888-82-4DADS
web site: www.dadsanddaughters.org

Daughters Magazine
Hoos Communications
8400 Fairway Place
Middleton, WI 53562
Tel: (615) 297-4778
Fax: (615) 297-9129
e-mail: daughters1@aol.com

Father Hunger: Fathers, Daughters and Food. Margo Maine. California: Gürze Books, 1991.

Growing Up Sad: Childhood Depression and Its Treatment. Leon Cytryn and Donald McKnew. New York: Norton, 1996.

I'm Not Mad, I Just Hate You! A New Understanding of Mother-Daughter Conflict. Roni Cohen-Sandler and Michelle Silver. New York: Viking, 1999.

New Moon Network: For Adults Who Care about Girls (newsletter)

Available from:
New Moon Publishing
PO Box 3587
Duluth, MN 55803-3587
(218) 728-5507

Raising a Daughter: Parents and the Awakening of a Healthy Woman. Jeanne Elium and Don Elium. California: Celestial Arts, 1994.

Reviving Ophelia: Saving the Selves of Adolescent Girls. Mary Pipher, PhD. New York: Ballantine Books, 1994.

Working Fathers: New Strategies for Balancing Work and Family. James Levine. New York: Addison-Wesley, 1997.

Puberty and Sexuality

Changes in You & Me: A Book about Puberty Mostly for Girls. Paulette Bourgeois & Martin Wolfish, MD. Toronto: Somerville House, 1994.

Speaking of SEX: Are You Ready to Answer the Questions Your Kids Will Ask? Meg Hickling. Kelowna, BC: Northstone Publishing, 1996.

The "What's Happening to My Body?" Book for Girls (1988); *The "What's Happening to My Body?" Book for Boys* (1988); *My Body, Myself* (1993). Lynda Madaras. New York: Newmarket Press.

Food

Becoming Vegetarian: The Complete Guide to Adopting a Healthy Vegetarian Diet. V. Melina, V. Harrison and B. Davis. Toronto: Macmillan, 1994.

The Enlightened Eater: A Guide to Well-Being through Eating. Rosie Schwartz. Toronto: Macmillan, 1998.

Full and Fulfilled: The Science of Eating to Your Soul's Satisfaction. Crossings, 1999.

The Nutrition Challenge for Women. Louise Lambert-Lagace. Toronto: Stoddart, 1989.

Working with Groups to Explore Food and Body Connections. Sandy Stewart Christian, ed. Duluth, MN: Whole Person Associates, 1996.

Diets and Weight

Making Peace with Food: Freeing Yourself from the Diet/Weight Obsession. Susan Kano. New York: Harper & Row, 1989.

When Women Stop Hating Their Bodies: Freeing Yourself from Food and Weight Obsession. Jane R. Hirschmann and Carol H. Munter. New York: Fawcett Columbine/Ballantine, 1995.

Why Weight: A Guide to Ending Compulsive Eating. Geneen Roth. New York: Plume, 1989.

Our Bodies

Body Wars: Making Peace with Women's Bodies (An Activist Guide). Margo Maine, PhD. California, Gürze Books, 1999.

My Body, My Rules: The Body Esteem, Sexual Esteem Connection (Resource and Activity Guide). Maureen Kelly.

Available from:
Planned Parenthood of Tompkins County
314 West State Street
Ithaca, NY 14850
(607) 273-1526 (ext. 126)

The New Our Bodies Ourselves. Boston Women's Health Collective. New York: Simon & Schuster, 1992.

Real Gorgeous: The Truth about Body and Beauty. Kaz Cooke. NSW, Australia: Allen & Unwin, 1994.

Transforming Body Image: Learning to Love the Body You Have. Marcia Germaine Hutchinson, ed. Freedom, CA: Crossing Press, 1985.

Sports and Physical Activity

The Bodywise Woman: Reliable Information about Physical Activity and Health. The Melpomene Institute. Englewood Cliffs, NJ: Prentice Hall, 1990.

Little Girls in Pretty Boxes: The Making and Breaking of Elite Gymnasts and Figure Skaters. Joan Ryan. New York: Doubleday, 1995.

On the Move: Increasing Participation of Girls and Women in Physical Activity and Sport. An initiative designed to encourage non-active teenage girls to participate in a fun-filled, supportive, low-skill level, team recreational activity. (This handbook is the result of a pilot project carried out in different parts of Canada.)

Available from:
Promotion Plus
#305-1367 West Broadway Street
Vancouver, BC V6H 4A9
Tel: (604) 737-3075
Fax: (604) 738-7175
web site: http://virtualplanet.com/promo_plus/

The Overweight Child: Promoting Fitness and Self-Esteem. Teresa Pitman and Miriam Kaufman, M.D. Toronto: Firefly Books, 2000.

Women's Sports Foundation
Eisenhower Park
East Meadow, NY 11554
Tel: (516) 542-4700
Fax: (516) 542-4716
e-mail: wosport@aol.com

Friends and Relationships

Best Friends: The Pleasures and Perils of Girls' and Women's Friendships. Teri Apter and Ruthellen Josselson. New York: Crown, 1998.

Dating Violence: Young Women in Danger. Barry Levy, ed. Seattle: Seal Press, 1991.

Where You and I Begin. Anne Catherine. New York: Fireside Books, 1993.

School

The AAUW Report: How Schools Shortchange Girls. The American Association of University Women Educational Foundation. Washington, DC: AAUW and National Education Association, 1992.

Failing at Fairness: How Our Schools Cheat Girls. Myra Sadker and David Sadker. New York: Simon & Schuster, 1994.

SchoolGirls: Young Women, Self-Esteem and the Confidence Gap. Peggy Orenstein (in association with the AAUW). New York: Doubleday, 1994.

Sounds from the Heart: Learning to Listen to Girls. Maureen Barbieri. Portsmouth, NH: Heinemann, 1995.

Bullying and Sexual Harassment

Battling the Schoolyard Bully: How to Raise an Assertive Child in an Aggressive World. Kim Zarzour. Toronto: Firefly Books, 2000.

Classrooms and Courtrooms: Facing Sexual Harassment in K-12 Schools. Nan Stein. New York: Teachers College Press (Columbia University), 1999.

Secrets in Public: Sexual Harassment in Our Schools. Nan Stein, Nancy L. Marshall and Linda R. Tropp. Wellesley, MA: NOW Legal Defense and Education Fund, and Wellesley College Center for Research on Women, 1993.

Available from:
Wellesley College Center for Research on Women
Wellesley, MA 02181-8259
(617) 283-2510

Sexual Harassment: High School Girls Speak Out. June Larkin. Toronto: Second Story Press, 1994.

Sexual Harassment and Teens: A Program for Positive Change. Susan Strauss. Minneapolis: Free Spirit Publishing, 1988.

Available from:
Free Spirit Publishing
400 First Avenue North, Suite 616
Minneapolis, MN 55401
(612) 338-1156

Media

GO GIRLS (Giving Our Girls Inspiration and Resources for Lasting Self-Esteem).

Available from:
EDAP (Eating Disorders Awareness and Prevention)
603 Stewart Street, Suite 803
Seattle, WA 98101
Tel: (206) 382-3587
Fax: (206) 829-8501
(Toll free) 1-800-931-2237
web site: www.edap.org.

Screen Smarts: A Family Guide to Media Literacy. Gloria DeGaetano and Kathleen Bander. Boston: Houghton Mifflin, 1996.

Where the Girls Are: Growing Up Female with the Mass Media. Susan J. Douglas. New York: Random House, 1994.

Resources for Girls

Are You Too Fat, Ginny? Karin Jasper. Toronto: IS Five Press, 1988.

Brave New Girls: Creative Ideas to Help Girls Be Confident, Healthy and Happy. (Money-related ideas and exercises.) Jeannette Gadeberg. Fairview Press, 1997.

The Creative Journal for Teens. Lucia Capacchione. California: Newcastle Publishing, 1992.

Depression Is the Pits, but I'm Getting Better: A Guide for Adolescents. E. Jane Garland. Washington, DC: Magination Press, 1997.

Girl Pages: A Handbook of the Best Resources for Strong, Confident, Creative Girls. Charlotte Milholland. Hyperion Books, 1998.

New Moon: The Magazine for Girls and Their Dreams (for girls 8 to 12).

Subscriptions from:
New Moon Publishing
P.O. Box 3587
Duluth, MN 55803-3587
(218) 728-5507

Period. JoAnn Gardner-Loulan, Bonnie Lopez and Marcia Quackenbush. California: Volcano Press, 1991.

The Seventeen *Guide to Sex and Your Body*. Sabrina Solin with Paula Elbert, MD. New York: Aladdin Paperback, 1996.

Tune Into Your Rights: A Guide for Teenagers about Turning Off Sexual Harassment. Eleanor Linn.

Available from:
Programs for Educational Opportunity
1005 School of Education
University of Michigan
Ann Arbor, MI 48109-1259
(313) 763-9910

A Very Touching Book. Jan Hindman. Oregon: AlexAndria Associates, 1983.

Social Action

DADS AND DAUGHTERS (DADs)
PO Box 3458
Duluth, MN 55803
(Toll free): 1-888-82-4DADS
web site: www.dadsanddaughters.org

Girls Incorporated
30 East 33rd Street
New York, NY 10016
Take Your Daughter to Work™ Day

Available from:
Ms. Foundation for Women
Dept. P, 141 Fifth Avenue
New York, NY 10016

Videos

Beyond the Looking Glass. 28 minutes. Grades 8-10 teacher resource (could be used for younger girls). Focuses on self-esteem, thoughts, feelings, identification of attitudes, stereotypes, body image. Provides direction to garner support for problem solving.

Available from:
Beyond the Looking Glass
41 Kensico Drive
Mt. Kisco, NY 10549
1-900-431-2050

Body Image (1998). 30 minutes. Video is designed to separate media hype from reality; to help young people make the right choices and develop an effective, healthy lifestyle.

Available from:
Heartland Releasing
1102-8th Avenue, 3rd floor
Regina, SA S4R 1C9
Tel: (306) 777-0888
Fax: (306) 586-3537

The Famine Within. Katherine Kilday (1990). 60 or 120 minutes. Ages 8-15. Explores the obsession with thinness and prejudice against fat. Reviews what dieting does to individuals.

Available from:
McNabb and Connolly
60 Briarwood Avenue
Port Credit, ON L5G 3N6
Tel: (905) 278-2801
Fax: (905) 278-0566

Killing Us Softly: Advertising's Image of Women (1979). 30 minutes. Produced by Cambridge Documentary Films. American feminist Jean Kilbourne casts a critical eye on the power and influence of advertising.

Still Killing Us Softly (1987). 30 minutes. Produced by Cambridge Documentary Films. This sequel to *Killing Us Softly* offers tools for developing a critical approach to mass media.

Slim Hopes: Advertising and the Obsession with Thinness. 30 minutes. Produced by Jean Kilbourne.

Available from:
Media Education Foundation
26 Center Street
Northampton, MA 01060

Take Another Look. 24 minutes. Produced by Lisa O'Brien and Bernice Vanderlaan. Dramatic fantasy on self-esteem for viewers aged 11-13. It encourages discussion on self-esteem, body image, the beauty and diet industries, self-respect and the need for peer support.

Available from:
McNabb and Connolly
60 Briarwood Avenue
Port Credit, ON L5G 3N6
Tel: (905) 278-2801
Fax: (905) 278-0566

Bibliography

American Association of University Women Educational Foundation. *The AAUW Report: How Schools Shortchange Girls*. Washington, DC: The AAUW Educational Foundation and National Education Association, 1992.

_____. *Shortchanging Girls, Shortchanging America*. Washington, DC, 1990.

_____. *Hostile Hallways: The AAUW Survey on Sexual Harassment in America's Schools*. Researched by Harris/Scholastic Research (division of Louis Harris and Associates) in partnership with Scholastic Inc. Washington, DC: The AAUW Educational Foundation, 1993.

American Journal of Health Promotion, 1996, Vol. 10.

Bassoff, Evelyn. *Mothers and Daughters: Loving and Letting Go*. New York: Plume, 1989.

Beauvoir, Simone de. *The Second Sex*, 2nd ed. H.M. Parshley, trans. New York: Vintage Books, 1972.

Berg. F. "Who Is Dieting in the United States?" *Obesity and Health*, May/June 1992.

Berger-Sweeney, Joanne. "The Developing Brain: Genes, Environment and Behavior." AAAS Symposium, February 9, 1996.

Block, Jeanne H. "Personality Development in Males and Females: The Influence of Differential Socialization." Paper presented as part of the Master Lecture Series at a meeting of the American Psychological Association, New York, September 1979.

Blum, Deborah. *Sex on the Brain: The Biological Differences between Men and Women.* New York: Viking, 1997.

Bruch, Hilde. *Eating Disorders: Obesity, Anorexia Nervosa and the Person Within.* New York: Basic Books, 1973.

Chapman, Gwen, and Heather Maclean. "'Junk Food' and 'Healthy Food': Meanings of Food in Adolescent Women's Culture." *Journal of Nutritional Education,* 1993, No. 25.

Colton and Gore. "Risk, Resiliency and Resistance: Current Research on Adolescent Girls." Ms. Foundation, 1991.

Cooke, Kaz. *Real Gorgeous: The Truth about Body and Beauty.* NSW, Australia: Allen & Unwin, 1994.

Dahlgren, Wendy. *A Report of the National Task Force on Young Females and Physical Activity.* Ottawa: Department of Fitness and Amateur Sport, 1988.

Douglas, Susan J. *Where the Girls Are: Growing Up Female with the Mass Media.* New York: Random House, 1994.

Eagle, Carol J., and Carol Colman. *All That She Can Be: Helping Your Daughter Achieve Her Full Potential and Maintain Her Self-Esteem during the Critical Years of Adolescence.* New York: Simon & Schuster, 1993.

Eichler, Margrit. *Families in Canada Today.* Toronto: Gage, 1983.

Elium, Jeanne, and Don Elium. *Raising a Daughter: Parents and the Awakening of a Healthy Woman.* California: Celestial Arts, 1994.

Erikson, Erik. *Identity, Youth and Crisis.* New York: W.W. Norton, 1968.

Featherstone, Heather. "Girls' Math Achievement: What We Do and Don't Know." *The Harvard Education Letter,* January 1986.

Feldman, W., E. Feldman and J. Goodman. "Health Concerns and Health Related Behaviour of Adolescents." *Canadian Medical Association Journal,* 1986, No. 134.

Fisher, William A., Donna Bryne and Leonard A. White. "Emotional Barriers to Contraception." In *Adolescents, Sex and Contraception.* Hillsdale, NJ: Lawrence Erlbaum, 1983.

Freud, Sigmund. *A General Introduction to Psychoanalysis.* J. Riviere, trans. New York: Permabooks, 1953.

Friedman, Sandra S. *Just for Girls Facilitator's Manual.* Vancouver: Salal Books, 1999.

Gilligan, Carol, and Lyn Mikel Brown. *Meeting at the Crossroads: Women's Psychology and Girls' Development.* Cambridge: Harvard University Press, 1992.

Gorney, Cynthia. "Teaching Johnny the Appropriate Way to Flirt." *New York Times Magazine,* June 13, 1999.

Gudykunst, William B., Stella Ting-Toomey, Sandra Sudsweeks and Lea P. Stewart, *Building Bridges: Interpersonal Skills for a Changing World.* Boston: Houghton Mifflin, 1995.

Hancock, Emily. *The Girl Within.* New York: Ballantine Books, 1989.

Health and Welfare Canada. *Nutrition Recommendations: The Report of the Scientific Review Committee.* Ottawa: Supply and Services, 1990.

Hickling, Meg. *Speaking of SEX: Are You Ready to Answer the Questions Your Kids Will Ask?* Kelowna, BC: Northstone Publishing, 1996.

Hirschmann, Jane R., and Carol H. Munter. *When Women Stop Hating Their Bodies: Freeing Yourself from Food and Weight Obsession.* New York: Fawcett Columbine/Ballantine Books, 1995.

Hutchison, Michael. *The Anatomy of Sex and Power: An Investigation of Mind-Body Politics.* New York: William Morrow, 1990.

Jasper, Karin. "Messages from the Media." Toronto: National Eating Disorder Information Centre Bulletin, March 1994, Vol. 9, No. 1.

Journal of the National Cancer Institute, 1994.

Kano, Susan. *Making Peace with Food: Freeing Yourself from the Diet/Weight Obsession.* New York: Harper & Row, 1989.

Kaplan, Alexandra G., Nancy Gelason and Rona Klein. "Women's Self Development in Late Adolescence." In Judith Jordon, Alexandra G. Kaplan, Jean Baker Miller, Irene P. Stiver and Janet L. Surrey, *Women's Growth in Connection: Writings from the Stone Center.* New York: Guilford Press, 1991.

Lajoie, Gesele, Alyson McLellan and Cindi Seddon. *Take Action against Bullying.* Coquitlam, BC: Bully Beware Productions, 1997.

Lamb, M.E., A. Frodi, C. Hwang, M. Frodi and J. Steinberg. "The Effects of Gender and Caretaking Role on Parent-Infant Interactions." In R. Emde and R. Harmon, eds., *Development of Attachment and Affiliation Systems.* New York: Plenum, 1982.

Larkin, June. *Sexual Harassment: High School Girls Speak Out.* Toronto: Second Story Press, 1994.

Larkin, June, Carla Rice and Vanessa Russell. "Slipping through the Cracks: Sexual Harassment, Eating Problems and the Problem of Embodiment." In *Eating Disorders: Journal of Treatment and Prevention*, Vol. 4, No. 1, Spring 1996.

Levy, Barrie, ed. *Dating Violence: Young Women in Danger.* Seattle: Seal Press, 1991.

MacInnis, Beth. "Fat Oppression." In Catrina Brown and Karin Jasper, eds., *Consuming Passions: Feminist Approaches to Weight Preoccupation and Eating Disorders.* Toronto: Second Story Press, 1993.

Madaras, Lynda. *The "What's Happening to My Body?" Book for Girls.* New York: Newmarket Press, 1988.

Maine, Margo. *Father Hunger: Fathers, Daughters and Food.* California: Gürze Books, 1991.

Medicine and Science in Sports and Exercise, 1996. Vol. 27.

Moe, Barbara. *Coping with Eating Disorders.* New York: Rosen Publishing Group, 1991.

Moir, Anne, and David Jessel. *Brain Sex: The Real Difference between Men and Women.* New York: Bantam, Doubleday Dell, 1991.

Offord, D., M.H. Boyle, P. Szatmari, et al. "Ontario Child and Health Study II: Six Month Prevalence of Disorder and Rates of Service Utilization." *Archives of General Psychiatry*, 1987, Vol. 44.

On the Move: Increasing Participation of Girls and Women in Physical Activity and Sport. Vancouver, BC: Premier's Sports Awards Program, 1993.

Orenstein, Peggy. *SchoolGirls: Young Women, Self-Esteem and the Confidence Gap*. New York: Doubleday, 1994.

Paplia, Diane E., and Sally Wendkos Olds. *A Child's World: Infancy through Adolescence*. New York: McGraw Hill, 1990.

Pediatric Exercise Science, 1994, Vol. 6.

Piesman, Marissa. *Heading Uptown: A Nina Fishman Mystery*. New York: Delacorte Press, 1993.

Pipher, Mary. *Reviving Ophelia: Saving the Selves of Adolescent Girls*. New York: Ballantine Books, 1994.

Pitman, Teresa, and Miriam Kaufman. *The Overweight Child: Promoting Fitness and Self-Esteem*. Toronto: Firefly Books, 2000. (Originally published as *All Shapes and Sizes* (HarperCollins).)

Reinisch, June M. "Fetal Hormones, the Brain and Human Sex Differences: A Heuristic Integrative Review of the Recent Literature." *Archives of Sexual Behavior*, 1974, No. 3.

Rubin, Z.R., E.J. Provenzano and Z. Luria. "The Eye of the Beholder: Parents' Views on the Sex of Newborns." *American Journal of Orthopsychiatry*, 1974, No. 44.

Ryan, Joan. *Little Girls in Pretty Boxes: The Making and Breaking of Elite Gymnasts and Figure Skaters*. New York: Doubleday, 1995.

Sadker, Myra, and David Sadker. *Failing at Fairness: How Our Schools Cheat Girls*. New York: Simon & Schuster, 1994.

Schieffelin, B., and E. Ochs. *Language Socialization across Cultures*. New York: Cambridge University Press, 1986.

Shakeshaft, C. "A Gender at Risk." *Phi Delta Kappan*, March 1986, Vol. 67, No. 7.

Sheldon, Amy. "Pickle Fights: Gendered Talk in Preschool Disputes." In Deborah Tannen, ed., *Gender and Conversational Interaction*. New York: Oxford University Press, 1993.

Siegler, Andria. "Grieving the Lost Dreams of Thinness." In Catrina Brown and Karin Jasper, eds., *Consuming Passions: Feminist Approaches to Weight Preoccupation and Eating Disorders*. Toronto: Second Story Press, 1993.

Smith, C., and B. Lloyd. "Maternal Behavior and Perceived Sex of Infant: Revisited." *Child Development*, 1978, No. 49.

Stein, Nan, Nancy L. Marshall and Linda R. Tropp. *Secrets in Public: Sexual Harassment in Our Schools*. Wellesley, MA: Center for Research on Women, Wellesley College, and the NOW Legal Defense and Education Fund, 1993.

Steinberg, Laurence, and Jay Belsky. *Infancy, Childhood and Adolescence: Development in Context*. New York: McGraw Hill, 1991.

Stiver, Irene P. "Beyond the Oedipus Complex: Mothers and Daughters." In Judith Jordan, et al., *Women's Growth in Connection: Writings from the Stone Center*. New York: Guilford Press, 1991.

Strauss, Susan. *Sexual Harassment and Teens: A Program for Positive Change*. Minneapolis: Free Spirit Publishing, 1988.

Surrey, Janet L. "The Self-in-Relation: A Theory of Women's Development." In Judith Jordan, et al., *Women's Growth in Connection: Writings from the Stone Center*. New York: Guilford Press, 1991.

Tannen, Deborah. *Talking from 9 to 5: How Men's and Women's Conversational Styles Affect Who Gets Heard, Who Gets Credit and What Gets Done at Work*. New York: William Morrow, 1994.

———. *You Just Don't Understand: Women and Men in Conversation*. New York: Ballantine Books, 1990.

Tenzer, S. "Fat Acceptance Therapy." In L. Brown and E. Rothblum, eds., *Overcoming Fear of Fat*. New York: Harrington Park, 1989.

U.S. Department of Health. *Youth Risk Behavior Survey*. 1990.

U.S. Department of Health and Human Services. *Report of the Surgeon General: Physical Activity and Health*. 1996.

Whiting, B., and C. Edwards. *Children of Different Worlds*. Cambridge: Harvard University Press, 1988.

Women's Sports Foundation Report: Sport and Teen Pregnancy. May 1998.

Wooley, S., and O. Wooley. "Obesity and Women: A Closer Look at the Facts." *Women's Studies International Quarterly*, 1979, No. 2.

Worthington-Roberts, B.S., and S.R. Williams, eds. *Nutrition through the Life Cycle*. St. Louis: Mosby, 1996.

Index

Visit the author at her web site:
www.salal.com

You can contact the author directly at:
salal@salal.net